MCQs
Basic Medica
for MRCP Part 1

D0864647

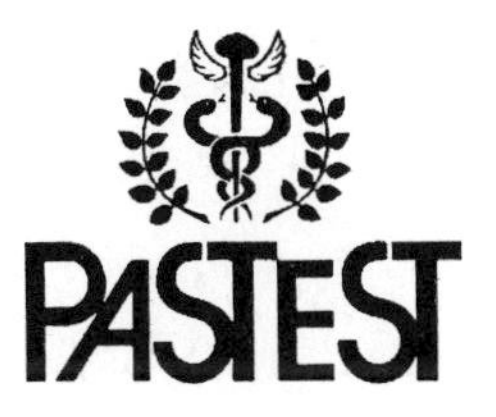

MCQs in Basic Medical Sciences for MRCP Part 1

Philippa J Easterbrook
MB BChir MRCP MPH MD
Senior Lecturer and
Consultant Physician in Infectious Diseases,
Chelsea and Westminster Hospital,
Charing Cross and Westminster Medical School,
London

Kefah M Mokbel
MB BS FRCS
Academic Surgical Unit,
Imperial College School of Medicine,
St Mary's Hospital,
London

© 1996 PASTEST
Knutsford
Cheshire
Telephone: 01565 755226

All rights reserved. No part of this publication may be reproduced, stored in a retrieval system, or transmitted, in any form or by any means, electronic, mechanical, photocopying, recording or otherwise without the prior permission of the copyright owner.

First edition 1996

ISBN: 0 906896 34 7

A catalogue record for this book is available from the British Library.

The information contained within this book was obtained by PasTest from reliable sources. However, while every effort has been made to ensure its accuracy, no responsibility for loss, damage or injury occasioned to any person acting or refraining from action as a result of information contained herein can be accepted by the publishers or authors.

Typeset by **EDITEXT**, Knutsford, Cheshire.
Printed by Hobbs The Printers Ltd, Totton, Hampshire.

CONTENTS

Correct answers and teaching notes follow the questions in each chapter.

PASTEST COURSES FOR MRCP PART 1

For over 22 years PasTest has been delivering top quality courses which have helped many thousands of doctors to pass the demanding MRCP Part 1 examination.

PasTest MRCP Part 1 courses are

- ✔ Intensive, practical and exam oriented
- ✔ Designed to strengthen exam technique
- ✔ Interactive and entertaining
- ✔ The key to exam success

Our reputation is built on results. With the official Royal College pass rate at 35%, PasTest delegates consistently achieve a pass rate of well over 60%. This is a competitive edge that you cannot afford to ignore.

Our popular six-day MRCP Part 1 revision courses run three times each year at convenient venues in London, Manchester, Dublin, Bristol and Stirling. There are also linked weekend (four-day) courses for those who cannot obtain study leave. Each delegate receives detailed course notes consisting of approximately 250 pages of exam-based MCQs with answers and comprehensive notes, plus many explanatory handouts.

- ✔ Learn from experienced and talented tutors with up-to-date knowledge of the requirements of the exam

- ✔ Teaching sessions focus on 'favourite' exam topics and highlight possible areas of difficulty

- ✔ Four full practice exams enable you to monitor your performance constantly as the course progresses

For full details of the range of PasTest books and courses available for MRCP Part 1 candidates, contact PasTest today:

PasTest, Dept. BSB, Egerton Court, Parkgate Estate,
Knutsford, Cheshire WA16 8DX
Telephone 01565 755226 Fax 01565 650264
E-mail pastest@dial.pipex.com

INTRODUCTION

This book is the result of a need for an MCQ revision guide on the basic medical sciences for MRCP Part 1. The current Royal College of Physicians MRCP regulations state:

> *Increased emphasis is being given to basic clinical science topics. Questions will be set mainly on topics published in leading articles and editorials in general medical journals. Questions in both options may be set on relevant principles of cell, molecular and membrane biology and immunology, genetics, and on biochemistry, as well as anatomical, physiological, microbiological and pharmacological topics.*

Thus this book has been written for all those who need help in tackling the basic medical sciences for Part 1 and also for Part 2 since candidates are now also examined frequently in the Part 2 viva on their understanding of the pathophysiology of disease processes, or on new developments in molecular medicine.

This book contains approximately 300 MCQs spanning the areas of genetics, molecular medicine, microbiology, immunology, anatomy, physiology, clinical chemistry, statistics and epidemiology, and clinical pharmacology. The chapter on clinical pharmacology focuses mainly on drug-induced disease and drug interactions – common recurring topics in the MRCP Part 1 exam. Most of the answers are extended to provide helpful background information beyond the points covered in the question.

The companion guide, *Basic Medical Sciences for MRCP Part 1* by Philippa Easterbrook, published by Churchill Livingstone (1st edition 1994) may serve as a helpful preliminary revision guide before attempting the MCQs in this book. In addition, the reader is encouraged to supplement his or her knowledge from the books and journal articles listed in the reference list.

I wish to thank Dr Kevin Talbot, MRC Training Fellow, University of Oxford, who contributed the chapter on molecular medicine, and the various MRCP candidates who previewed the material. Finally, I am grateful to Jane Bowler at PasTest for her skill and forbearance during the production of this book.

I hope this book will be both stimulating and helpful for candidates preparing for the examination and I would be interested to hear of any errors or ambiguities that readers encounter when working through this book.

PJE
London, 1996

The multiple choice questions which appear in this book are based on the most recent MRCP Part 1 examination papers and are designed to cover a wide range of relevant basic science topics. Each question consists of an initial statement (or 'stem') followed by five possible completions (or 'items') identified by A, B, C, D or E. There is no restriction on the number of true or false items in a question. It is possible for all items in a question to be true or for all to be false. The four most important points of technique are:

1. Read the question carefully and be sure you understand it.
2. Mark your response clearly, correctly and accurately.
3. Use reasoning to work out your answer, but if you do not know the answer and cannot work it out, indicate 'Don't know'.
4. The best possible way to obtain a good mark is to have as wide a knowledge as possible of the topics being tested in the examination.

To get the best value from this book you should commit yourself to an answer for each item before you check the correct answer. Mark your answers in the boxes provided next to each item. To calculate your score, give yourself a mark for each correct item, and subtract a mark for each incorrect item. Items marked 'Don't know' score zero.

You must read the question (both stem and items) carefully. You should be quite clear that you know what you are being asked to do. Once you know this, you should indicate your response by marking the paper boldly, correctly and clearly. In an official examination take great care not to mark the wrong boxes and think very carefully before making a mark on the computer-marked answer sheet.

Regard each item as being independent of every other item – each refers to a specific quantum of knowledge. The stem and item taken together make up a statement. You are required to indicate whether you regard this statement as true or false, and you are also able to indicate 'Don't know'. Look only at a single statement when answering – disregard all the other statements presented in the question, they have nothing to do with the one you are concentrating on.

Since the answer sheet will be read by a computer it must be filled out in accordance with the instructions. As you go through the questions you can either mark your answers immediately on the answer sheet, or mark them in the question book in the first instance, and then transfer them to the answer sheet at the end. In view of the time pressure you may be best advised to mark your answers directly onto the answer sheet as you go along. Put a clear mark next to any questions you found particularly difficult so that you can quickly find them again if you have time to review them at the end of the exam.

Candidates are frequently uncertain whether or not to guess the answer. Experience shows that you should back your hunches. Only if you are completely in the dark should you record a 'Don't know' answer. Thus, if the question gives you a clue or your knowledge is sufficient to give you a hunch about the correct answer, you will probably gain from guessing.

All too often candidates' marks suffer through an inability to organise their time or through failure to read the instructions carefully. You must ruthlessly allocate your time during the examination. In MRCP Part 1 there are 60 questions to complete in 2½ hours, that is 2½ minutes per question or 10 questions in 25 minutes. Make sure that you are getting through the exam at this pace or a little quicker to allow time at the end to look through your answers.

Tips for Revision in the Basic Medical Sciences for MRCP Part 1

Revision needs to be geared to the examination you are sitting. It should confirm the areas you know well and consolidate the areas where your understanding is unfocused. An important part of revision is the identification of areas where the work required will *not* result in sufficient gain to justify the time.

WHAT YOU SHOULD DO	WHAT YOU SHOULD NOT DO
* Integrate basic sciences with clinical topics.	* Attempt to study major text books or original articles on basic science.
* Concentrate on recurring examination themes and topical issues.	* Concentrate on topics you like and understand in too much detail.
* Remember the structure and format of the MRCP Part I questions.	* Study controversial or unresolved issues.

RECOMMENDED READING AND REFERENCE BOOKS

Basic Medical Sciences for MRCP Part 1
P Easterbrook
Churchill Livingstone, 1st edition 1994

Essential Medical Genetics
J M Connor, M A Ferguson-Smith
Blackwell Scientific Publications, 4th edition 1993

Alberts Molecular Biology of the Cell
Garland, 3rd edition 1994

Microbiology in Clinical Practice
D C Shanson
Butterworth Heinemann, 2nd edition 1995

Essentials of Clinical Immunology
H Chapel, M Haeney
Blackwell Scientific Publications, 3rd edition 1993

Clinical Anatomy
H Ellis
Blackwell Scientific Publications, 8th edition 1991

Review of Medical Physiology
W F Ganong
Appleton & Lange, 16th edition 1995

Textbook of Medical Physiology
A C Guyton
Saunders, 9th edition 1990

Biochemistry
L Stryer
Freeman, 4th edition 1995

Clinical Epidemiology: The Essentials
R H Fletcher, S W Fletcher, E H Wagner
Williams & Wilkins, 3rd edition 1995

Introduction to Medical Statistics
M Bland
Oxford University Press, 2nd edition 1995

Clinical Pharmacology
D R Laurence, P N Bennett
Churchill Livingstone, 7th edition 1992

Suggested articles on topical issues for review

Special articles, review articles and leading articles in the *New England Journal of Medicine, Lancet* and *BMJ* periodically cover topical issues. I would not recommend reading all (or even most) of these but dipping into two or three may clarify areas that you find confusing. The list is not meant to be comprehensive but does identify some of the themes covered in recent MRCP questions. Remember that the exam is set at least a year in advance – don't waste time reading last week's journals.

Nitric Oxide and Vascular Disease, J Loscalzo, *NEJM*, **333:** 251–253, 1995.

Oncogenes, T G Krontiris, *NEJM*, **333:** 303–306, 1995.

Endothelins, E R Levin, *NEJM*, **333:** 356–363, 1995.

The Primary Immunodeficiencies, F S Rosen et al., *NEJM*, Vol. **333:** 431–440, 1995.

Mitochondrial DNA and Disease, D R Johns, *NEJM*, **333:** 638–644, 1995.

Gene Therapy – A Novel Form of Drug Delivery, H M Blau and M L Springer, *NEJM*, **333:** 1204–1207, 1995.

Transcription Factors, A G Papavassiliou, *NEJM*, **332:** 45–47, 1995.

Regulation of Gene Expression, N Rosenthal, *NEJM*, **331:** 931–933, 1994.

Nitric Oxide: Mediator, Murderer and Medicine, E Anggard, *Lancet*, 343: 1199–1206, 1994.

Cancer Progression and p53, D A Carson and A Lois, *Lancet*, **346:** 1009–1011, 1995.

Pathogenesis of Multiple Sclerosis, C ffrench-Constant, *Lancet*, **343:** 271–275, 1994.

Haemolytic–Uraemic Syndrome, Basic Science and Practice, J L Moake, *Lancet*, **343:** 393–397, 1994.

Familial Cancer Syndrome, S C Eng et al., *Lancet*, **343:** 709–713, 1994.

Leucocyte–Endothelial Interactions and Regulation of Leucocyte Migration, D H Adams and S Shore, *Lancet*, **343:** 831–836, 1994.

Free Radicals, Antioxidants and Human Disease: Curiosity, Cause or Consequence? B Halliwell, *Lancet,* **344:** 721–724, 1994.

Hepatitis C Virus Six Years On, C L Van der Poel et al., *Lancet*, **344:** 1475–1479, 1994.

Alcoholic Liver Disease, S Sherlock, *Lancet*, **345:** 227–229, 1995.

Hypercoagulable States: Molecular Genetics to Clinical Practice, A I Schafer, *Lancet*, **344:** 1739–1742, 1994.

Tumour Suppressor Genes in Disease and Therapy, G R Skuse and J W Ludlow, *Lancet*, **345:** 902–906, 1995.

Aplastic Anaemia, N S Young, *Lancet*, **346:** 228–232, 1995.

Dr Donal O'Donoghue
Consultant Renal Physician
Hope Hospital, Salford.

1: GENETICS

Mark your answers with a tick (True) or a cross (False) in the box provided before checking against the correct solutions. Leave the box blank for 'Don't know'.

1. Autosomal dominant inheritance is present in

☐ A von Willebrand's disease
☐ B Duchenne muscular dystrophy
☐ C dystrophia myotonica
☐ D hereditary spherocytosis
☐ E galactosaemia

2. The following disorders are transmitted on the X-chromosome:

☐ A familial Mediterranean fever
☐ B glucose-6-phosphate dehydrogenase deficiency
☐ C haemophilia B
☐ D phenylketonuria
☐ E colour blindness

3. The following statements regarding autosomal recessive inheritance are true:

☐ A if an affected individual marries a normal person, then 50% of the children will be carriers
☐ B if husband and wife are both carriers, then 25% of the children will be carriers
☐ C there is a tendency to skip a generation
☐ D it occurs in cystic fibrosis
☐ E the disease is usually not as serious as a dominantly inherited one

4. Chromosome abnormalities are found in the following conditions:

☐ A Huntington's chorea
☐ B Klinefelter syndrome
☐ C myeloid leukaemia
☐ D achondroplasia
☐ E cri-du-chat disease

5. HLA-B8 associated diseases include

☐ A ankylosing spondylitis
☐ B myasthenia gravis
☐ C multiple sclerosis
☐ D coeliac disease
☐ E dermatitis herpetiformis

6. The following relatives of a haemophiliac may manifest disease:

☐ A father
☐ B mother
☐ C sisters
☐ D father's brother
☐ E mother's brother

7. Screening is available routinely in the UK for the relatives of patients with the following:

☐ A Tay–Sachs' disease
☐ B Duchenne muscular dystrophy
☐ C Gilbert's disease
☐ D sickle cell disease
☐ E Wilson's disease

8. The following show autosomal recessive inheritance:

☐ A galactosaemia
☐ B Huntington's chorea
☐ C vitamin D resistant rickets
☐ D cystinuria
☐ E manic depressive illness

9. Which of the following traits or diseases are transmitted by a Mendelian dominant gene:

☐ A polyposis coli
☐ B tuberose sclerosis
☐ C haemophilia
☐ D congenital pyloric stenosis
☐ E neurofibromatosis

10. Turner's syndrome is associated with

☐ A ovarian agenesis
☐ B congenital absence of the uterus
☐ C adrenal hyperplasia
☐ D tumour of the ovary
☐ E virilizing tumour of the adrenal gland

11. Autosomal recessive traits

☐ A occur mainly in males
☐ B affected individuals usually have normal parents
☐ C both parents are heterozygous carriers of the genes
☐ D one quarter of the male and female children of two heterozygous parents will be affected
☐ E one quarter of the children will be heterozygous carriers for the trait

12. Klinefelter syndrome is associated with

- ☐ A azoospermia
- ☐ B increased incidence of breast cancer
- ☐ C chromatin positive nuclear pattern
- ☐ D reversible infertility
- ☐ E precocious puberty

13. In Turner's syndrome (46XO)

- ☐ A treatment with growth hormone may increase final height
- ☐ B there is an increased risk of gonadal neoplasia in the streak ovary
- ☐ C there is ambiguity of the external genitalia
- ☐ D the Mullerian structures are absent
- ☐ E there is an increased incidence of hypertension

14. The following are recognized features of Down's syndrome:

- ☐ A coarctation of the aorta
- ☐ B secundum atrial septal defect
- ☐ C early development of Alzheimer's disease
- ☐ D increased prevalence of atherosclerosis
- ☐ E deletion of chromosome 15q 11–13

15. The following statements about DNA structure are correct:

- ☐ A there are two purine bases called adenine (A) and thymidine (T)
- ☐ B guanine (G) always pairs with cytosine (C) and adenine (A) with thymidine (T)
- ☐ C an amino acid codon consists of three bases
- ☐ D each strand of DNA has a sugar-phosphate backbone with projecting bases
- ☐ E there are 132 possible codons

16. In a family with hypertrophic obstructive cardiomyopathy (HOCUM), the following statements are true:

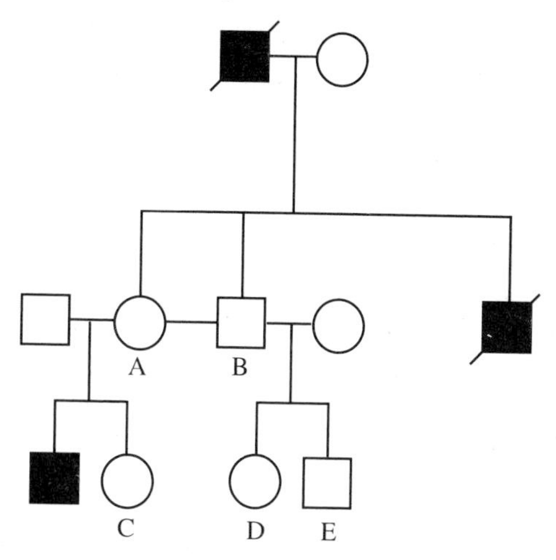

A the mode of transmission in the family is X-linked recessive inheritance
B echocardiography is an essential prerequisite to risk estimation and genetic counselling
C approximately 75% of individuals who carry the gene are symptomatic with dyspnoea on exercise and syncope
D beta-blockers are contraindicated
E For individuals D and E the risk of inheriting the disease is negligible

17. A patient's maternal serum alpha fetoprotein (AFP) is found to be elevated above the 97th percentile on a routine ante-natal sample at 17 weeks' gestation. The following statements are correct:

A if the amniotic fluid AFP is also elevated, the possibilities include twins, or threatened abortion
B it may be a normal finding if the amniotic fluid AFP is normal
C amniocentesis is indicated for measurement of amniotic fluid AFP after a second abnormal result
D amniotic fluid acetyl cholinesterase isoenzymes can be used to confirm the diagnosis of a neural tube defect
E approximately 10% of children born with neural tube defects have mothers with no family history of the disorder

ANSWERS AND TEACHING NOTES: GENETICS

The correct answer options are given against each question.

1. A C D

Duchenne muscular dystrophy is inherited in a **sex-linked recessive** fashion. Galactosaemia inheritance is autosomal recessive.

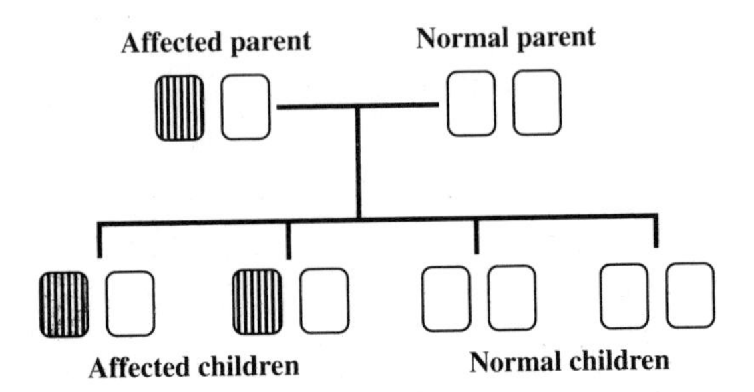

The following diseases are inherited in an **autosomal dominant** manner:

α_1 anti-trypsin deficiency
achondroplasia
acute intermittent porphyria (also variegate porphyria)
adult polycystic kidney disease
Ehlers–Danlos syndrome
facioscapulohumeral dystrophy
Gilbert's syndrome
hereditary spherocytosis
Huntington's chorea
hyperlipidaemia type II
malignant hyperthermia
Marfan's syndrome
myotonia congenita
myotonic dystrophy
neurofibromatosis
Noonan syndrome
osteogenesis imperfecta (some forms)
polyposis coli
rotor syndrome
retinoblastoma gene
tuberosis sclerosis
von Willebrand's disease

2. B C E

Sex-linked inheritance occurs in more than 1000 conditions, e.g. colour blindness, haemophilia A and B, Duchenne muscular dystrophy, Becker's dystrophy. Familial Mediterranean fever is an autosomal recessive condition and phenylketonuria is inherited in an autosomal recessive fashion.

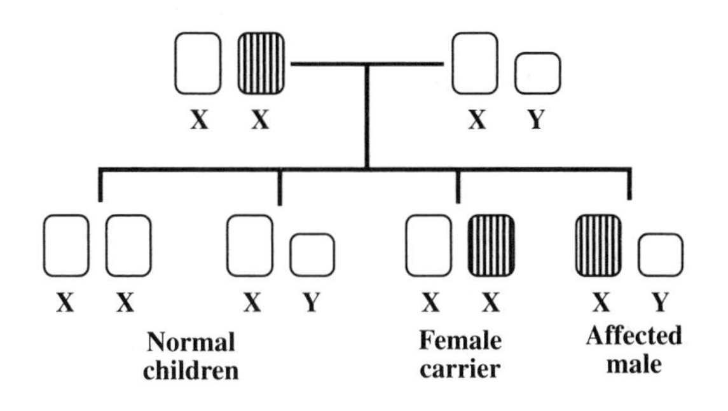

The following are inherited in an **X-linked** fashion:

agammaglobulinaemia
Becker's muscular dystrophy
chronic granulomatous disease
colour blindness
complete testicular feminization
Duchenne muscular dystrophy
Fabry's disease
glucose-6-phosphate dehydrogenase deficiency
haemophilia A (factor VIII deficiency)
haemophilia B (factor IX deficiency)
Hunter's syndrome
ichthyosis (steroid sulphatase deficiency)
Lesch–Nyhan syndrome (hypoxanthine guanine phosphoribosyl transferase deficiency)
nephrogenic diabetes insipidus
ocular albinism
retinitis pigmentosa
Wiskott–Aldrich syndrome
(NB Vitamin D resistant rickets is X-linked dominant.)

3. C D

If an affected person marries a normal person, then all children will be carriers. If the husband and wife are carriers then 50% of the offspring will be carriers. Autosomal recessive disease is usually more serious than a dominantly inherited condition.

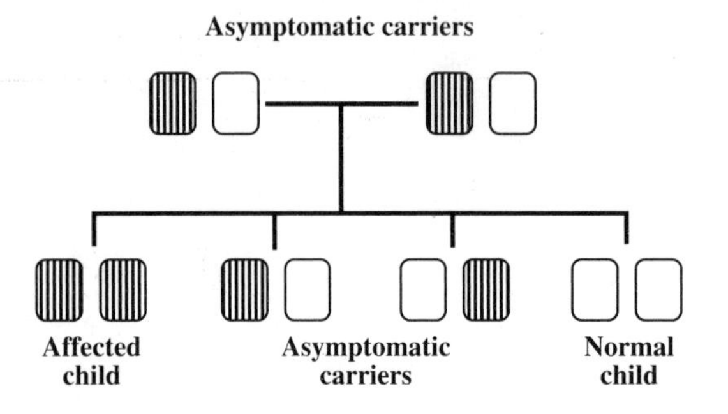

The following are **autosomal recessive** conditions:

albinism
ataxia telangiectasia
congenital adrenal hyperplasia
Crigler–Najjar syndrome type I
cystinuria
cystic fibrosis
deafness (some forms)
Dubin–Johnson syndrome
familial Mediterranean fever
Fanconi's anaemia
Friedreich's ataxia
galactosaemia
Gaucher's disease
glycogen storage diseases
haemochromatosis
homocystinuria
Hurler syndrome
limb girdle muscular dystrophy (Erb)
Niemann–Pick disease
Pendred's syndrome
phenylketonuria
sickle cell disease

Tay–Sachs' disease
thalassaemias
Wilson's disease

4. **B C E**

The frequency of chromosome abnormalities at birth is approximately 5.6 per 1000. Of these, about 2 per 1000 are due to a variation in the number of sex chromosomes, 1.7 per 1000 are due to a variation in numbers of autosomal chromosomes, and 1.9 per 1000 are major chromosomal rearrangements. These abnormalities account for 60 or more different clinical conditions. Among the commoner and best defined are Down's syndrome (trisomy 21), Edwards' syndrome (trisomy 18), Patau syndrome (trisomy 13), Klinefelter syndrome (sex chromosomes XXY) and Turner's syndrome (XO monosomic sex disorder). The Philadelphia chromosome is an acquired chromosomal abnormality present in 85% of cases of chronic myeloid leukaemia, due to the deletion of the long arm of chromosome 22 with translocation, usually on to chromosome 9. The 'cri du chat' syndrome is due to a partial deletion of the short arm of chromosome 5. Achondroplasia has an autosomal dominant pattern of inheritance.

5. **B D E**

The haplotype B8, DR3 is particularly common in organ-specific disorders where cell-surface antigens are prime targets. In Graves' disease and myasthenia gravis these have been identified as TSH and ACH receptors respectively. B8 is also in linkage disequilibrium with DR3 (i.e. it occurs with DR3 more often than expected by chance). Conditions associated with HLA B8 include dermatitis herpetiformis, insulin-dependent diabetes, thyrotoxicosis, Addison's disease, coeliac disease, chronic active hepatitis, myasthenia gravis and Sjogren's with Sicca syndrome.

6. **E**

Haemophilia is transmitted by carrier women who produce affected boys, normal boys, carrier girls and normal girls with equal frequency. Affected cases have affected brothers and maternal uncles, and can only have normal sons and carrier daughters. (See the answer to Question 2.)

7. A B D E

In the UK, carrier screening is only undertaken for haemoglobinopathies, Tay–Sachs' disease, thalassaemia and sickle cell disease. However, screening can be performed, if available, for Duchenne muscular dystrophy and Wilson's disease.

8. A D

Huntington's chorea has an autosomal dominant pattern of inheritance. Vitamin D resistant rickets has X-linked dominant inheritance. Manic depressive illness has a polygenic inheritance. (See the answer to Question 3.)

9. A B E

Haemophilia A and B have a sex-linked recessive inheritance, and congenital pyloric stenosis has a polygenic inheritance. (See the answer to Question 1.)

10. A

Turner's syndrome (karyotype 45XO) is characterized by a phenotypic female, short stature, wide carrying angle, webbing of neck, short metacarpals, sexual infantism, primary amenorrhoea, high gonadotrophin levels, low oestrogen levels and slight intellectual defect. Associated anomalies include coarctation of the aorta and renal abnormalities.

11. B C D

In autosomal recessive inheritance, both sexes are equally affected. Asymptomatic carriers produce affected children. When both parents carry the gene, 1 in 4 children are affected, and 2 in 4 children are carriers. (See the answer to Question 3.)

12. A B C

Klinefelter syndrome (karyotype 47XXY, XXXYY or XXYY) is characterized by tall, thin men with bilateral gynaecomastia and infertility due to hypogonadism, high urinary gonadotrophins and an increased incidence of mental subnormality. Patients present with defective sexual maturation and have an increased incidence of breast cancer and a slight predisposition to germ cell tumours compared with other males. The infertility is irremediable.

13. A E

Large doses of growth hormone result in increased final height if treatment is started sufficiently early. An increased risk of gonadal dysplasia applies only to gonadal dysgenetic syndromes where there is a Y chromosome (for example, 46XY pure gonadal agenesis). Immature Mullerian structures are present. The increased risk of hypertension is caused by essential hypertension, coarctation of the aorta or renal abnormalities.

14. B C

The most common heart defects in Down's syndrome are atrioventricular canal defects (40% compared with 2–3% in the normal population), secundum atrial septal defect and patent ductus arteriosus. Aortic stenosis and coarctation of the aorta are rare. Nearly all Down's syndrome patients have some evidence of Alzheimer's disease by the time they are 40 years old. There is decreased prevalence of atherosclerosis in Down's syndrome, although the reasons for this are not clear. Deletion of chromosome 15q 11–13 is typical of the Prader–Willi syndrome. Trisomy 21 is the classical chromosomal abnormality in Down's syndrome.

15. B C D

There are two purine bases called adenine (A) and guanine (G) and two pyrimidine bases called thymidine (T) and cytosine (C). G always pairs with C and A with T. An amino acid codon consists of three bases. As each base in the triplet may be any of the four types of nucleotide (A, G, C, T) this results in 64 possible codons. Most amino acids have more than one codon and some codons signal chain termination.

16. B

HOCUM usually shows an autosomal dominant transmission. The male to male transmission in this family tree rules out an X-linked recessive inheritance. In this condition, expression is very variable and only 25% of carriers of the disease genes are symptomatic. Characteristic echocardiographic abnormalities in those with the HOCUM gene include asymmetric ventricular septal hypertrophy, and echocardiography is therefore a prerequisite to genetic counselling. Symptoms may develop at any age and include fatigue, dyspnoea on exercise, angina pectoris and syncope. The prognosis is highly variable, but about 75% of individuals who carry the gene are asymptomatic and have a normal life span. Beta-blockers may be effective. Individuals B and C had a 1 in 2 chance of inheriting the disease, and for D and E, the risk is about 17%.

17. B C D

The causes of elevated maternal serum alpha fetoprotein can be divided into two groups:

1. Normal amniotic fluid AFP:
   - normal finding (top 3% of the distribution);
   - wrong dates;
   - twins;
   - threatened abortion;
   - maternal hereditary persistence of AFP.

2. Elevated amniotic fluid AFP:
   - encephaly;
   - open spina bifida;
   - anterior abdominal wall defect;
   - congenital nephrotic syndrome;
   - and fetal skin defects.

The test may be offered to any mother who has previously had an affected child. However, about 90% of children born with neural tube defects have mothers with no family history of the disorder. The maternal serum AFP should be repeated and ultrasound examination performed to check the gestation, exclude twins, and look for neural tube defects. If ultrasound examination is normal and a second serum AFP is elevated, amniocentesis is indicated for measurement of amniotic fluid AFP and banding.

2: MOLECULAR MEDICINE

1. Endothelin

- ☐ A is a circulating vasoregulatory substance in man
- ☐ B causes bronchospasm
- ☐ C is produced from a precursor under the regulation of angiotensin converting enzyme
- ☐ D has been implicated in the pathogenesis of pulmonary hypertension
- ☐ E is raised in the serum of patients with essential hypertension

2. Nitric oxide

- ☐ A synthesis is stimulated by TNF (tumour necrosis factor)
- ☐ B is likely to be a useful therapy in angina
- ☐ C is inhibited by the lipopolysaccharide of Gram-negative bacteria
- ☐ D is a neurotransmitter
- ☐ E exists in a free radical form which can be neurotoxic

3. Interleukin-1

- ☐ A cannot be detected in individuals in the absence of inflammation
- ☐ B blood levels are a useful index of disease activity in rheumatoid arthritis
- ☐ C infused intravenously leads to hypotension
- ☐ D is a neurotransmitter
- ☐ E antagonizes the effect of tumour necrosis factor

4. Protooncogenes

- ☐ A are carcinogenic retroviruses
- ☐ B are only expressed in malignant tissues
- ☐ C control cell growth and differentiation
- ☐ D are transiently upregulated by growth factors
- ☐ E inactivate oncogenes

5. Tumour suppressor genes

- ☐ A exert a recessive effect genetically
- ☐ B include the gene which causes neurofibromatosis type I
- ☐ C act to switch the cell into mitosis
- ☐ D include the p53 protein
- ☐ E are viral in origin

6. G-proteins

- ☐ A are activated by the exchange of GDP for GTP
- ☐ B include ras oncoproteins
- ☐ C are mutated in pituitary adenomas
- ☐ D are transmembrane signal receptor molecules
- ☐ E are found in all cell types

7. Apoptosis

- ☐ A causes necrotic cell death
- ☐ B is involved in embryonic remodelling
- ☐ C releases proinflammatory mediators
- ☐ D is characterized by condensation of nuclear chromatin
- ☐ E is associated with endonuclease activity

8. Tumour necrosis factor

- ☐ A causes cachexia
- ☐ B is produced by bronchogenic carcinoma
- ☐ C is likely to be a useful therapy for rheumatoid arthritis
- ☐ D is elevated in septic shock
- ☐ E kills tumour cells *in vitro*

9. Transforming growth factor β

- ☐ A promotes wound healing
- ☐ B is released from platelets during degranulation
- ☐ C stimulates protease activity
- ☐ D has autocrine activity
- ☐ E stimulates lymphocyte proliferation

10. p53

- ☐ A supresses cell division
- ☐ B is a viral protein
- ☐ C mutation promotes tumour growth
- ☐ D has a normal function in developmental control
- ☐ E is required for apoptosis of cells in which DNA has been damaged

11. Regarding malignancy

- ☐ A malignant cells die by apoptosis
- ☐ B resistance to drugs may be conferred by mutant genes
- ☐ C mutation of the p53 gene is an adverse prognostic marker
- ☐ D most tissues can be shown to demonstrate cytogenetic abnormalities
- ☐ E the inherited tendency to the development of cancer always follows a Mendelian pattern

12. In the polymerase chain reaction (PCR)

- ☐ A several thousand copies of the target sequence are required for successful amplification
- ☐ B Guthrie blood spot cards can be used to perform retrospective genetic diagnosis
- ☐ C DNA fragments up to one megabase can be successfully amplified
- ☐ D RNA as well as DNA can be used in PCR
- ☐ E analysis of genetic abnormalities using a single cell can be performed

13. Monoclonal antibodies

☐ A are mouse antibodies
☐ B can be used in medical imaging
☐ C are likely to be useful therapeutic agents because they have no side effects
☐ D are manufactured by using transgenic animals
☐ E are not in themselves immunogenic

14. The following statements about cellular signal transduction are true:

☐ A all signal transduction requires the coupling of G-proteins to a second messenger
☐ B glucocorticoids bind directly to DNA
☐ C second messenger systems allow amplification of an external stimulus
☐ D insulin receptors are ligand gated ion channels
☐ E the acetylcholine receptor is a chloride channel

15. Trinucleotide DNA repeats

☐ A are the molecular explanation for the phenomenon of genetic anticipation
☐ B are unstable in somatic mitosis
☐ C are the cause of the Fragile X syndrome
☐ D cause Duchenne muscular dystrophy
☐ E can produce a polyglutamine peptide sequence which has been implicated in neurodegeneration

16. Prion diseases

☐ A are caused by retroviruses
☐ B include Alzheimer's disease
☐ C are unique in that genetic forms can be passed on to laboratory animals by injection of affected brain material
☐ D include scrapie in sheep
☐ E are caused by a protein that is resistant to the action of proteases

17. Steroid hormone receptors

- ☐ A are located on the cell surface membrane
- ☐ B when activated bind DNA
- ☐ C are functionally similar to thyrotrophin receptors
- ☐ D are transcription factors
- ☐ E are mutated in some breast cancers

18. The following statements are true of interferons:

- ☐ A interferon-γ inhibits macrophage killing
- ☐ B interferon-β has a more potent antiviral effect than interferon-γ
- ☐ C interferon-β treatment decreases the number of demyelinating plaques on MRI in multiple sclerosis
- ☐ D interferons have structural similarity to the immunoglobulin superfamily of molecules
- ☐ E interferon-β and interferon-γ act at the same receptors

19. Mitochondrial DNA

- ☐ A contains no introns
- ☐ B is inherited exclusively from the mother
- ☐ C mutations can cause diabetes mellitus
- ☐ D shows variation from cell to cell within the same individual
- ☐ E contains the genes for the enzymes of glycolysis

20. The following molecules are paired with their correct function:

- ☐ A integrins are involved in complement mediated cell lysis
- ☐ B heat shock proteins function as molecular chaperones in the export of protein within cell organelles
- ☐ C vitamin B2 is a principal dietary source of antioxidant
- ☐ D ras is a guanine nucleotide binding protein
- ☐ E dystrophin is a form of nerve growth factor

ANSWERS AND TEACHING NOTES: MOLECULAR MEDICINE

1. B D

Endothelins are a family of structurally similar 21 amino acid peptides. Endothelin-1 is the most potent vasoconstrictor substance yet described. It is produced following vascular endothelial 'stress' (for example, shear, hypoxia, growth factors, expansion of plasma volume) from pre-pro endothelin by the action of ETCE (endothelin converting enzyme). The function of endothelin is as a paracrine (i.e., acting on neighbouring cells) regulator of vascular tone and blood pressure, and circulating levels of the hormone are not relevant to disease processes or normal homoeostasis. There are receptors for endothelin on vascular endothelium and on smooth muscle cells in the gut and the lung. Mutations in the endothelin B receptor are one cause of Hirschsprung's disease and it therefore has a role in the embryonic development of neural crest tissue.

Clinical relevance: Endothelin has been implicated in the pathogenesis of

- chronic heart failure
- essential hypertension
- hepatorenal syndrome
- primary pulmonary hypertension
- Raynaud's phenomenon
- renovascular hypertension
- vasospasm after subarachnoid haemorrhage

2. A D E

Nitric oxide (NO) is a gas and an important transcellular messenger molecule, which is synthesized from the oxidation of nitrogen atoms in the amino acid L-arginine by the action of NO synthase (NOS). NO acts on target cells close to its site of synthesis where it activates guanylate cyclase leading to a rise in intracellular cyclic guanosine monophosphate (GMP) which acts in turn as a second messenger to modulate a variety of cellular processes. It has a very short half-life, and is broken down rapidly in the circulation to nitrates and nitrites. The expression of NO is controlled by the distribution of NOS which has a constitutive (i.e., produced at a basal level) isoform active in brain (mediating memory formation) and vascular endothelium (causing vasodilatation). It also has an inducible form in mononuclear phagocytes (part of the innate immune response activated by cytokines and involved in the killing of micro-organisms). NO is also a free radical which can interact with other reactive oxygen species to lead to lipid peroxidation of cell membranes and subsequent cell death. Synthetic nitrates, such as glyceryl trinitrate and sodium nitroprusside, act after their conversion into NO.

Clinical relevance:

atherosclerosis
(where loss of NO-dependent vasodilatation leads to vasospasm)
cell death in the CNS
hypotension in septic shock
pulmonary hypertension

3. C

Interleukin-1β has a broad spectrum of both beneficial and harmful biological actions and is a central regulator of the inflammatory response. It is synthesized by activated mononuclear phagocytes and secreted into the circulation where it is cleaved by interleukin-1β converting enzyme (ICE).

Clinical relevance:

In septic shock interleukin-1 (IL-1) acts by increasing the concentration of small mediator molecules, such as PAF (platelet activating factor), prostaglandins and nitric oxide, which are potent vasodilators.
IL-1 is present in the synovial lining and fluid of patients with rheumatoid arthritis and it is thought to activate gene expression for collagenases, phospholipases and cyclooxygenases. Serum levels are not relevant to disease activity.
IL-1 has some host defence properties, inducing T and B lymphocytes and reduces mortality from bacterial and fungal infection in animal models.

4. C D

Oncogenes were originally identified as genes carried by cancer causing viruses. They are the mutated form of normal genes called protooncogenes, that are usually highly conserved in evolution and have central roles in the signal-transduction pathways that control cell growth and differentiation in eukaryotes. Examples of the range of cellular processes affected are given below:

Classification	Example	Function
Growth factors	*sis*	platelet-derived growth factor
Growth factor receptors	*trk*	receptor for nerve growth factor
Intracellular transducers	*ras*	G-protein
Nuclear transcription factors	*myc*	DNA binding protein

Only one mutated copy of the gene is required to promote malignant growth as, by definition, the mutation of the gene leads to activation.

5. A B D

Tumour supressor genes, in contrast to oncogenes, exert a recessive effect, in that two 'hits' are required before loss of function and tumorigenesis occur. Several types of inherited cancers involve this mechanism, e.g. the NF-1 gene product 'neurofibromin'. These genes normally function to inhibit the cell cycle and therefore when inactivated lead to loss of growth control. p53 is a protein which occupies a pivotal role in the cell cycle and is the most commonly mutated gene in tumours (e.g. breast and colon). It encodes a transcription factor which downregulates the cell cycle and therefore prevents cells from entering mitosis.

6. A B C E

Membrane bound receptors which are binding sites for an external stimulus or first messenger (e.g. light, hormones, neurotransmitters) interact with second messenger pathways that are responsible for ultimately leading to a change in the state of the cell, for example, a growth factor binding to a cell surface receptor leads to initiation of mitosis and cell division. The coupling of first and second messengers via G-proteins is an ubiquitous and fundamental mechanism in biology. G-proteins are typically composed of three subunits (α, β and γ). When a ligand binds to its receptor, the alpha subunit of the G-protein then releases GDP and binds GTP which gives it an active conformation that allows it to interact with a second messenger system, such as cyclic-GMP. G-proteins control many cellular processes, such as neurotransmission, cell division and hormone action.

Clinical relevance:

Pseudohypoparathyroidism, where there is generalized resistance to a variety of hormones. The dysmorphic features are due to a reduction in the activity of the G-protein that activates adenylatecyclase in response to hormones, such as PTH, T3 and gonadotrophins.

Cholera: *Vibrio cholerae* secretes an exotoxin that makes a G-protein resistant to inactivation and this ultimately leads to fluid and electrolyte loss.

Mutations activating G-proteins occur in about 40% of patients with acromegaly.

7. B D E

Apoptosis describes the morphological changes (shrinkage, chromatin condensation and phagocytosis) seen when cells undergo programmed cell death. This is a genetically regulated mechanism for removing unwanted cells both in embryological development (e.g. more than 50% of motor neurones die in embryological life) and during adult life both in health (e.g. the removal of autoreactive lymphocytes) and disease (e.g. loss of CD4 positive lymphocytes in AIDS). In contrast to inflammation, apoptosis does not lead to the release of potentially damaging intracellular contents (e.g. free radicals or proteases) into the surrounding milieu. Cancer can be seen in part as a failure of apoptosis; the oncogene *bcl-2* inhibits cells from entering programmed cell death.

8. A D E

Tumour necrosis factor (TNF) is an important proinflammatory cytokine with actions that are similar and complementary to IL-1 in initiating and sustaining the inflammatory response. There are two forms of TNF which bind to the same receptors but are coded for by separate genes. TNF-α is produced by activated mononuclear phagocytes, NK cells and eosinophils. TNF-β is produced by activated T-lymphocytes. The name TNF derives from the observation that it can kill tumour cells directly in culture but this is probably not its primary function *in vivo*.

Clinical relevance:

overproduction of TNF has been implicated in causing wasting, mediating septic shock in response to Gram-negative endotoxin and in autoimmune disorders (anti-TNF antibodies are beneficial in rheumatoid arthritis).

9. A B D

Transforming growth factor β (TGF-β) is a key cytokine and growth factor that initiates and terminates tissue repair and whose sustained production underlies the development of tissue fibrosis. It acts by binding to specific cell surface receptors which are present on most cell types. The response of a particular cell to TGF-β depends on the presence of other growth factors and the cell type. It has a potent effect on cells to induce the production of extracellular matrix (a dynamic superstructure of self-aggregating macromolecules, including fibronectin, collagen and proteoglycans, to which cells attach by means of surface receptors called integrins). Extracellular matrix is continually being degraded by proteases which are inhibited by TGF-β. TGF-β is released by platelets at the site of tissue injury and is strongly chemotactic for monocytes, neutrophils, T cells and fibroblasts. It induces monocytes to begin secreting FGF (fibroblast growth factor), TNF and IL-1, but inhibits the functioning of T and B cells and their production of TNF and IL-1. It also induces its own secretion. This autoinduction may be important in the pathogenesis of fibrosis.

Clinical relevance:

> Elevated plasma levels of TGF-β are highly predictive of hepatic fibrosis in bone marrow transplant recipients. mRNA for TGF-β is found in areas of active disease in the liver biopsies of patients with chronic liver disease. In patients with idiopathic pulmonary fibrosis, TGF-β is increased in the alveolar walls. TGF-β is likely to be used as an agent to promote wound healing and bone repair.

10. A C D E

p53 is a protein coded for by a tumour supressor gene which occupies a pivotal role in the cell cycle and is the most commonly mutated gene in tumours (e.g. breast, colon). It encodes a transcription factor the normal function of which is to downregulate the cell cycle by preventing the cell from entering mitosis. It is the primary defect in the Li–Fraumeni syndrome (a familial cancer syndrome involving the development of multiple solid organ tumours) and is a central regulator of apoptosis.

11. A B C D

Cancer cells are a clonal population of cells in which the accumulation of mutations in multiple genes has resulted in escape from the normally strictly regulated mechanisms which control growth and differentiation of somatic cells. Cancer is thus a multistep process and although examples of pure inherited cancer syndromes due to one mutant gene occur they are not the cause of most solid tumours which are more usually attributed to a varying degree of interaction between heredity and environment. As tumours grow they become more bizarre in their growth (showing a high degree of cytogenetic abnormalities) and accumulate more mutations which in turn allows them to escape the effect of cytotoxic drugs. Damaged cells normally undergo apoptosis under the regulation of the p53 protein, but p53 mutations allow cancer cells to survive toxic insults, such as radiotherapy. However, those cancer cells that die do so by programmed cell death using pathways other than p53.

12. B D E

In the polymerase chain reaction (PCR), DNA which contains a target sequence to be amplified is mixed with oligonucleotide primers (typically 20–30 base pairs in length) and a special heat-stable DNA polymerase derived from a micro-organism (*T. aquaticus*) which lives in hot springs. PCR is a way of amplifying a specific region of DNA to produce many copies that can be analysed to detect the presence of specific gene sequences or markers. Its applications in medicine are numerous and include the detection of viral sequences in tissue samples (e.g. herpes simplex DNA in the CSF in encephalitis) and the diagnosis of specific mutations in genetic diseases and cancer. It is theoretically possible to produce enough DNA by PCR amplification for analysis using only one cell but in practice at least 10–100 molecules are needed as a template. RNA can also be used as a template when it has been converted to complementary DNA (cDNA) by reverse transcriptase. With standard techniques the limit of template size that can be amplified is around 2–3kb.

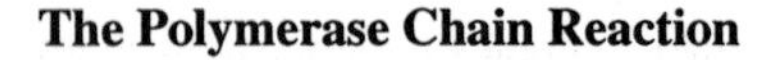

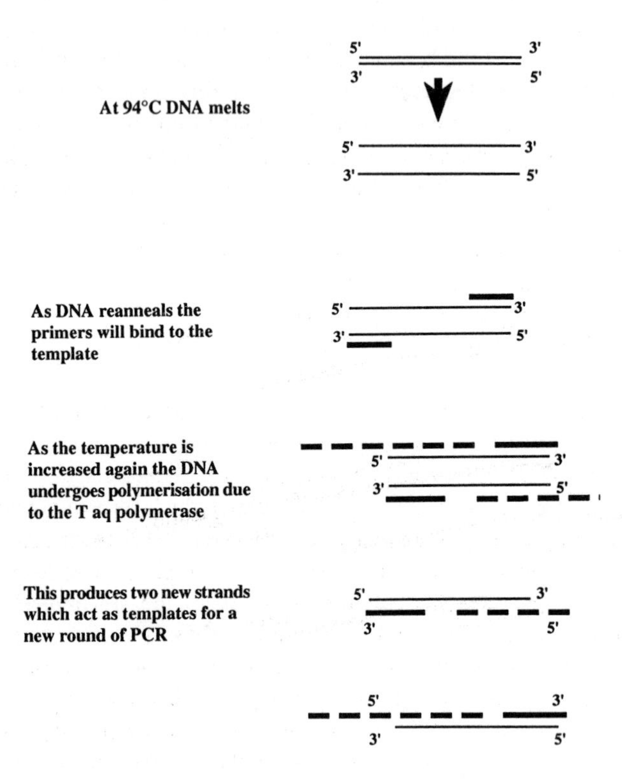

13. A B

Monoclonal antibodies are highly specific mouse antibodies which can be produced in large amounts and have found a wide range of applications in medicine. Myeloma is a malignantly transformed B-cell lineage which secretes a specific antibody. This observation is used to produce specific antibodies directed toward an antigen of interest. A laboratory animal, following injection with an antigen of choice, mounts an immune response and its spleen is then harvested. The cells are fused *en masse* to a specialized myeloma cell line which no longer produces its own antibody (this avoids the production of cells which secrete two types of antibody). The resulting fused cells, or hybridomas, constitute an immortalised cell line, and produce antibodies specified by the lymphocytes of the immunized animal. These cells can be screened to select for the antibody of interest which can then be produced in unlimited quantity. Human anti-mouse antibodies (HAMAs) produced by recipients of mouse monoclonals have limited their usefulness. In order to circumvent this problem monoclonal antibodies can be 'humanised' by joining the antigen binding site from the mouse antibody to the constant region of human antibodies, thereby retaining specificity while limiting cross-species antigenicity.

Clinical applications:

diagnosis of cancer and infections
imaging of tumours and radiotherapy
aim to use as 'magic bullet' to direct anti-rejection drugs
in transplantation and other immune modulators

14. C

Although G-proteins are a very common way of connecting first messengers to second messenger systems this is not the only method used by cells for signal transduction. For example, lipophilic molecules, such as steroids, pass through the cell membrane to interact directly with cytosolic receptors. Many neurotransmitters are the ligand for ion channels, such as the acetylcholine receptor, which is a sodium channel. Some membrane receptors act by direct enzymatic activation of second messengers without the use of G-proteins, but most of these systems are characterized by an enormous degree of amplification (i.e. one first messenger leads ultimately to a cascade of activation of many intracellular molecules).

15. A B C E

A new class of genetic mutation has been recognized in recent years which is the cause of a number of important human genetic neurological diseases. Repeating units of three nucleotides (e.g. CAG, CTG, CGG) have been found in the coding and non-coding sequences of a number of genes. In most cases there is a variable number of repeats in the general population over a small range; that is, the number of repeats shows polymorphism. At the upper end of the range the stretch of repeats appears to become unstable during DNA replication and the number of repeats may undergo amplification. If this produces a long enough run of repeats the gene is disrupted and the disease becomes manifest. Because of the unstable nature of trinucleotide repeats, the size of the expansion may increase in successive generations. This provides a molecular explanation for the phenomenon of genetic anticipation where the offspring of a patient with Huntington's disease will generally develop the disease earlier and have a larger expansion than their parent. The triplet CTG codes for glutamine and this amino acid have been implicated in so-called 'excitoxic cell death' in the CNS. It has therefore been proposed that these polyglutamine peptide sequences produced by runs of CTG are in themselves neurotoxic.

Diseases caused by trinucleotide repeats include:

Fragile X mental retardation
Friedreich's ataxia and other hereditary ataxias
Huntington's disease
myotonic dystrophy

16. C D E

Diseases caused by prions in humans include Creutzfeldt–Jakob disease (CJD), Gerstmann–Straussler syndrome (GSS) and fatal familial insomnia. Affected individuals show spongiform change in the brain at necropsy with the accumulation of amyloidogenic protein. Prions (proteinaceous infective particles) are unique agents which appear to cause infectious disease without the transmission of nucleic acid (DNA or RNA) to the affected individual. The abnormal protein found in the brains of affected individuals has a normal cellular counterpart coded for by a gene (the human prion protein gene). It appears that the protein itself in its altered form can cause the disease by some novel mechanism. Furthermore, the disease has the potential to be both genetic and infectious. Ten per cent of cases of CJD and most cases of GSS show autosomal dominant inheritance and mutations of the prion protein gene. Yet the brain tissue of these patients with genetic disease can be injected into primates and will cause the disease after a long incubation period. Iatrogenic cases of CJD have occurred with the injection of pooled samples of human pituitary gland and the use of dura mater from necropsy specimens as neurosurgical patches.

17. B C D E

Although all cells contain the same complement of genes (genotype), a nerve cell is clearly different in its morphology and behaviour (phenotype) from a lymphocyte. It is the regulation of gene expression which underlies this difference. Genes are regulated by proteins called transcription factors which bind to specific regions of DNA (located near genes), called promoter and enhancer elements. Transcription factors therefore have specific DNA binding domains with recurrent structural motifs, which are the basis for their classification. For example, transcription factors with a 'helix–turn–helix' motif are important in developmental regulation in the embryo. The 'zinc finger' motif consists of pairs of amino acids which grasp a zinc atom and push a polypeptide out into a loop (finger) which binds specific regions of DNA. An example of this kind of transcription factor is the steroid hormone receptor. Steroids act by binding to a receptor which is part of a complex bound to intracellular cytosolic membrane. When the steroid hormone binds, this releases the hormone receptor complex which is able to bind to promoter elements on specific genes called 'hormone responsive elements'. Corticosteroids belong to a class of hormones called the 'nuclear hormone superfamily' which all act in this way. This class includes vitamin D, retinoic acid, oestrogens and thyroid hormone.

Clinical relevance:

Transcription factors can act as oncogenes when they are mutated to alter the expression of growth factors. Many hormones and drugs act at the level of transcription factors.

Transcription factors may be a suitable target for gene therapy experiments (e.g. the upregulation of fetal haemoglobin in sickle cell anaemia).

18. B C

Interferon-γ is produced by T-lymphocytes and NK cells in response to viral infection. It is an inhibitor of viral replication and mediates a host of other immunological functions, including the upregulation of MHC Class I and II expression and efficiency of macrophage mediated killing. IFN-γ binds to a specific receptor which is different from that of interferons-α,β and mediates its functions through the induction of a range of other molecules. The inhibition of viral replication by interferon is mediated by the production of a protein kinase which phosphorylates the active site of the initiation factor responsible for protein synthesis. Interferon-β is an immunomodulator which has been shown to reduce the MRI changes in multiple sclerosis.

19. A B C D

The mitochondrial genome is circular and approximately 16 kb in length. It encodes genes for the mitochondrial respiratory chain and for some species of transfer RNA. No mitochondria are transferred from spermatozoa at fertilization and so each individual only inherits mtDNA from the mother. Because there are thousands of mitochondria in each cell the mtDNA content of an individual will be heterogeneous. There is evidence that mtDNA mutations are accumulated throughout life and that this may contribute to the changes of ageing. Several diseases have been shown to be due to mtDNA mutations and these are mostly neurodegenerative diseases with a variable phenotype that can encompass lactic acidosis and diabetes.

20. B D

Integrins are heterodimeric transmembrane glycoproteins which are widely distributed in different tissues and serve to interact with molecules of the extracellular matrix (e.g. laminin, fibronectin, collagen).

The **heat shock response** is a highly conserved and phylogenetically ancient response to tissue stress that is mediated by activation of specific genes. This response leads to an alteration in transcription and the production of specific heat shock proteins that alter the phenotype of the cell. Their diverse functions include the export of proteins in and out of specific cell organelles (acting as molecular 'chaperones'), the catalysis of protein folding and unfolding and the degradation of proteins (often by the pathway of 'ubiquitination').

Antioxidant molecules are involved in the neutralization of oxygen based free radicals which damage cells by lipid peroxidation. The principal dietary source of antioxidants are vitamins A and C and beta carotene.

Ras stands for rat sarcoma virus and denotes a family of 21kD proteins (H, K and N) found on the cytoplasmic aspect of the plasma membrane. It is a G-protein, but of the 'small' monomeric subclass, and is therefore likely to be involved in transduction of growth promoting signals. At least a third of sporadic tumours contain acquired somatic mutations in ras.

Dystrophin is a very large muscle protein which is involved in anchoring the cell membrane and muscle cytoskeleton. Mutations in dystrophin lead to the X-linked progressive muscular dystrophies of Becker and Duchenne.

3: MICROBIOLOGY

1. ***Neisseria meningitidis***

- ☐ A has a polysaccharide capsule
- ☐ B infection is usually diagnosed by detecting serum antibodies
- ☐ C may cause the Waterhouse–Friderichsen syndrome
- ☐ D infection is transmitted by airborne droplets
- ☐ E vaccine is mainly composed of a group B polysaccharide capsule

2. ***Listeria monocytogenes***

- ☐ A is a Gram-negative rod
- ☐ B is an important cause of meningitis in the newborn
- ☐ C is usually treated with ciprofloxacin
- ☐ D can be transmitted through unpasteurized milk
- ☐ E can be effectively prevented by vaccination

3. ***Haemophilus influenzae***

- ☐ A is a Gram-positive rod
- ☐ B vaccine is unconjugated
- ☐ C organisms causing systemic infections are almost always encapsulated
- ☐ D is sensitive to amoxycillin
- ☐ E frequently causes urinary tract infections

4. Penicillin G is active against

- ☐ A *Neisseria meningitidis*
- ☐ B *Escherichia coli*
- ☐ C *Pseudomonas aeruginosa*
- ☐ D most anaerobic infections
- ☐ E *Klebsiella aerogenes*

5. The following causative viruses and associated diseases are correctly paired:

- ☐ A rotaviruses – Lassa fever
- ☐ B Coxsackie B – meningitis
- ☐ C flaviviruses – Ebola fever
- ☐ D HTLV-II – Hairy T-cell leukaemia
- ☐ E HTLV-I – adult T-cell leukaemia

6. The following features are characteristic of hepatitis B infection:

- ☐ A raised titres of anti-HBs occur during the incubation period of hepatitis B infection
- ☐ B hepatitis B virus is present in the saliva and semen of infected persons
- ☐ C the presence of anti-HBs in serum indicates immunity
- ☐ D the presence of 'e' antigen in serum indicates immunity
- ☐ E the risk of transmission with a needlestick injury from a HBsAg positive source is less than 5%

7. In human immunodeficiency virus (HIV) infection

- ☐ A seroconversion following HIV infection generally occurs 3–12 weeks following infection and is usually asymptomatic
- ☐ B there is no confirmed association between acquisition of HIV infection and history of sexually transmitted disease
- ☐ C progression to AIDS is associated with a fall in the CD4/CD8 ratio and beta-2-microglobulin levels
- ☐ D 50% of HIV infected individuals will develop AIDS within 10 years of infection
- ☐ E the membrane envelope of HIV contains two linked glycoproteins, p24 and p17

8. *Legionella pneumophila*

☐ A is a recognized cause of atypical pneumonia
☐ B infection is usually diagnosed by culturing sputum
☐ C infection is usually transmitted through person-to-person contacts
☐ D is sensitive to erythromycin
☐ E causes a rise in cold agglutinin titres

9. The following infections in pregnant women are known to cause defects in the fetus:

☐ A toxoplasmosis
☐ B mumps
☐ C rubella
☐ D infectious mononucleosis
☐ E measles

10. Patients with sickle cell disease are more prone to the following infections:

☐ A *Neisseria meningitidis*
☐ B *Haemophilus influenzae*
☐ C *Mycobacterium tuberculosis*
☐ D *Salmonella* species
☐ E Varicella zoster

11. The following statements are true concerning the congenital rubella syndrome:

☐ A the newborn child may develop a retinopathy
☐ B it carries the greatest risk to the fetus if the mother has rubella during the third trimester
☐ C in congenital infection the virus can be isolated from the throat of the newborn whether or not signs of the disease are present
☐ D coarctation of the aorta commonly occurs in the newborn
☐ E bony lesions may be seen on the X-ray of affected neonates

12. Specific contraindications to routine primary vaccination include

☐ A immunosuppressive therapy
☐ B infantile eczema
☐ C first trimester of pregnancy
☐ D under six months of age
☐ E during an epidemic

13. Congenital toxoplasmosis is characteristically associated with

☐ A the appearance of calcification on skull X-ray
☐ B involvement of neonates in successive pregnancies
☐ C congenital cardiac lesions if the fetus is affected in the first trimester
☐ D bilateral chorioretinitis
☐ E renal abnormalities

14. *Escherichia coli*

☐ A bears spores
☐ B is a non-lactose fermenter
☐ C does not grow well anaerobically
☐ D is a Gram-negative rod
☐ E is sensitive to tetracycline

15. The following features are characteristic of Creutzfeldt–Jakob disease:

☐ A human to human transmission
☐ B almost all cases are familial affecting mainly men
☐ C may be linked with bovine spongiform encephalography found in cattle
☐ D brain pathology reveals extensive inflammation and demyelination
☐ E characteristically a disease of late middle age (5th–7th decade of life)

16. The following infections may be acquired from contact with animals or animal products:

- ☐ A leptospirosis
- ☐ B tularaemia
- ☐ C plague
- ☐ D typhoid fever
- ☐ E brucellosis

17. Production of exotoxin is an important factor in the pathogenicity of

- ☐ A *Escherichia coli*
- ☐ B *Klebsiella* spp.
- ☐ C *Mycobacterium tuberculosis*
- ☐ D *Corynebacterium diphtheriae*
- ☐ E *Vibrio cholerae*

18. Bacterial pathogens that may be carried asymptomatically in the upper respiratory tract include

- ☐ A *Bordetella pertussis*
- ☐ B *Neisseria meningitidis*
- ☐ C *Haemophilus influenzae* type B
- ☐ D group A haemolytic streptococci
- ☐ E *Mycobacterium tuberculosis*

19. *Staphylococcus aureus* has a well-established association with

- ☐ A toxic epidermal necrolysis
- ☐ B cholecystitis
- ☐ C toxic shock syndrome
- ☐ D acute osteomyelitis
- ☐ E food poisoning

20. Characteristics of infections caused by *Staphylococcus aureus* resistant to beta-lactam antibiotics include

- ☐ A person-to-person transmission is the major route of spread
- ☐ B beta-lactam resistant isolates are less virulent than beta-lactam susceptible isolates
- ☐ C asymptomatic carriage in the nares or rectum of hospital staff is uncommon
- ☐ D beta-lactam resistant isolates are sensitive to methicillin
- ☐ E most strains are coagulase negative and catalase positive

21. The following vaccines may be given safely to individuals who are HIV antibody positive:

- ☐ A measles
- ☐ B hepatitis B
- ☐ C BCG
- ☐ D mumps
- ☐ E yellow fever

22. Hepatitis C virus (HCV)

- ☐ A is a DNA virus
- ☐ B may be transmitted parenterally
- ☐ C has a seroprevalence rate of 60–90% in haemophiliacs
- ☐ D rarely leads to chronic liver disease
- ☐ E may be treated effectively with high-dose acyclovir

23. ***Streptococcus pneumoniae***

- ☐ A has five different polysaccharide serotypes
- ☐ B is an important cause of subacute bacterial endocarditis
- ☐ C may become resistant to penicillin because of beta-lactamase production
- ☐ D causes clinical infection more readily in individuals with sickle cell disease
- ☐ E may be prevented from causing invasive disease in children less than 2 years old by vaccination

24. Parvovirus B19

- ☐ A is a DNA virus
- ☐ B is a recognized cause of diarrhoea in children
- ☐ C infection is frequently asymptomatic
- ☐ D causes erythema nodosum
- ☐ E causes aplastic crises in patients with haemolytic anaemia

25. ***Helicobacter pylori***

- ☐ A is a Gram-positive, flagellate bacillus
- ☐ B is found in the mucus that lines the gastric epithelium
- ☐ C is present in most patients with duodenal ulcer disease
- ☐ D is effectively eradicated by a two-week course of bismuth, metronidazole and tetracycline
- ☐ E should be eradicated in cases of gastric ulceration

26. The following antimicrobial drugs are effective against penicillinase-producing staphylococci:

- ☐ A ampicillin or amoxycillin
- ☐ B phenoxymethylpenicillin
- ☐ C cefuroxime
- ☐ D vancomycin
- ☐ E cloxacillin

27. *Enterococcus faecalis*

- ☐ A is highly susceptible to penicillin
- ☐ B is a cause of infective endocarditis
- ☐ C is included in the common term 'viridans streptococci'
- ☐ D possesses Lancefield group D carbohydrate antigen
- ☐ E is associated with food poisoning

28. The following clinical presentations or mechanisms are matched with the correct causative organism:

- ☐ A nausea, vomiting, diarrhoea and flaccid paralysis within 18–36 hours and food-borne botulinum toxin
- ☐ B nausea and vomiting within 1–6 hours and *Staphylococcus aureus* preformed enterotoxin
- ☐ C abdominal cramps and diarrhoea within 8–16 hours and *Bacillus cereus* enterotoxin production *in vivo*
- ☐ D paraesthesia within 1–6 hours and ciguatera fish poisoning
- ☐ E a toxin which increases the production of adenyl cyclase and enterotoxigenic *E. coli* (ETEC)

29. Common causes of diarrhoea among travellers to tropical areas are

- ☐ A enterotoxigenic *Escherichia coli*
- ☐ B enteroinvasive *Escherichia coli*
- ☐ C *Giardia lamblia*
- ☐ D *Entamoeba histolytica*
- ☐ E *Enterococcus faecalis*

30. *Cryptosporidium parvum* infection

- ☐ A can be acquired from contaminated water sources
- ☐ B a modified AFB smear of the stool may be a useful diagnostic test
- ☐ C outbreaks in day centres have been described
- ☐ D the causative organism may be easily killed by adequate chlorination of water supplies
- ☐ E causes a self-limiting diarrhoeal disease in immunocompromised patients

31. The following infecting pathogens are matched with the most appropriate therapeutic agent:

☐	A	*Strongyloides stercoralis*	thiabendazole
☐	B	*Fasciola hepatica*	praziquantel
☐	C	*Aspergillus fumigatus*	ketoconazole
☐	D	*Toxoplasma gondii*	primaquine
☐	E	*Onchocerca volvulus*	quinacrine

32. DNA may be transferred naturally among bacteria by

☐ A recombination
☐ B transduction
☐ C conjugation
☐ D transcription
☐ E mutation

33. Recombinant hepatitis B vaccine

☐ A is highly effective with approximately 90% protection
☐ B is a whole virus vaccine
☐ C offers some cross protection against hepatitis A
☐ D frequently causes arthritis is patients who already have antibodies against hepatitis surface antigen
☐ E has a lower response rate in patients with chronic liver disease

34. HIV is reliably inactivated by

☐ A hot air oven
☐ B glutaraldehyde
☐ C hypochlorites
☐ D autoclave
☐ E chlorhexidine

35. The following infections and transmission routes are correctly paired:

- ☐ A *T. cruzii* infection and exposure to contaminated fresh water lakes
- ☐ B Ebola virus and infected Rhesus monkeys
- ☐ C Katayama fever and *Aëdes* spp. mosquitoes
- ☐ D *Herpesvirus simiae* (B virus) and blood transfusions
- ☐ E *Leishmania tropica* and sandfly

36. The following flaviviruses may depend on human rather than vertebrate animal hosts in their primary transmission cycle:

- ☐ A Japanese encephalitis
- ☐ B tick-borne encephalitis
- ☐ C dengue fever
- ☐ D yellow fever
- ☐ E St Louis encephalitis

37. The following antiviral agents are correctly matched with the site of inhibition of viral replication:

☐	A zidovudine	reverse transcriptase
☐	B ganciclovir	uncoating of RNA in cell
☐	C amantadine	viral DNA polymerase
☐	D interferon	viral protein synthesis, assembly and release
☐	E stavudine	HIV protease

ANSWERS AND TEACHING NOTES: MICROBIOLOGY

1. **A C D**

   N. meningitidis is a Gram-negative diplococcus and has a polysaccharide capsule which can be detected in CSF by use of a latex agglutination test. *N. meningitidis* is usually considered to be part of the oropharyngeal flora and can be found in 20–40% of healthy young adults. During epidemics of meningococcal diseases in institutionalized populations, colonization rates may approach 90%. The meningococcal vaccine contains capsular polysaccharides of A, C, Y and W-135 strains. No vaccine is currently available for group B meningococci (responsible for 70% of cases of meningococcal septicaemia in the UK) because of the poor immunogenicity of their capsular polysaccharide.

2. **B D**

   The two most common agents of neonatal bacteraemia are *Listeria monocytogenes* and Group B streptococci. Both are Gram-positive diplococci and may be confused on Gram stain. They can easily be distinguished by the catalase test. *L. monocytogenes* is catalase positive, whereas group B streptococcus is catalase negative. Both are susceptible to ampicillin. Outbreaks of systemic infection following ingestion of contaminated food, usually dairy products, are well documented in pregnant women and immunocompromised patients. *Listeria monocytogenes* infections are usually self-limiting in the mother but can have devastating consequences for the child leading to stillbirth, septic abortion, premature delivery, pneumonia and meningo-encephalitis.

3. **C D**

   H. influenzae is a small Gram-negative, non-motile and non-sporing rod that may cause meningitis, sinusitis, pneumonia, otitis media and rarely, epiglottitis. The latter may cause upper airway obstruction. Chocolate agar provides abundant quantities of both factor X (hemin) and nicotinamide-adenine dinucleotide (factor V) – specific requirements for growth of *H. influenzae*. Organisms causing systemic infection are almost always encapsulated, and *H. influenzae* encapsulated with Type b polysaccharide accounts for over 90% of cases of bacteraemia. A protective conjugated vaccine (to increase immunogenicity and impove host antibody response) has been developed against *H. influenzae* Type b, coupled with either diphtheria or tetanus toxoid. This combination vaccine is now approved for use in infants with the initial series of vaccinations at 2, 4 and 6 months of age. Amoxycillin is used in the treatment and rifampicin in prophylaxis against *H. influenzae* meningitis.

4. A D

Penicillin is effective against most aerobic Gram-positive organisms. It is not effective against most Gram-negative rods, such as *H. influenzae, E. coli* and *P. aeruginosa*, though ampicillin and amoxycillin have some activity. Penicillin is also inactive against bacterial cells which are not growing.

5. B D E

Rotaviruses cause upper respiratory tract infections and infantile diarrhoea. Both Lassa fever and Ebola virus disease are due to arena viruses with a high person-to-person transmission and a relatively high case fatality rate. Flaviviruses cause yellow and dengue fevers.

6. B C

Appearance of anti-HBs in the serum usually signifies a successful recovery from infection. Clinical recovery and clearance of the virus is associated with disappearance of HBeAg and then HBsAg, with subsequent detection of their respective antibodies during recovery. 'e' antigen is a marker of infectivity. The risk of transmission with a needlestick injury from a HBsAg positive source is approximately 30%.

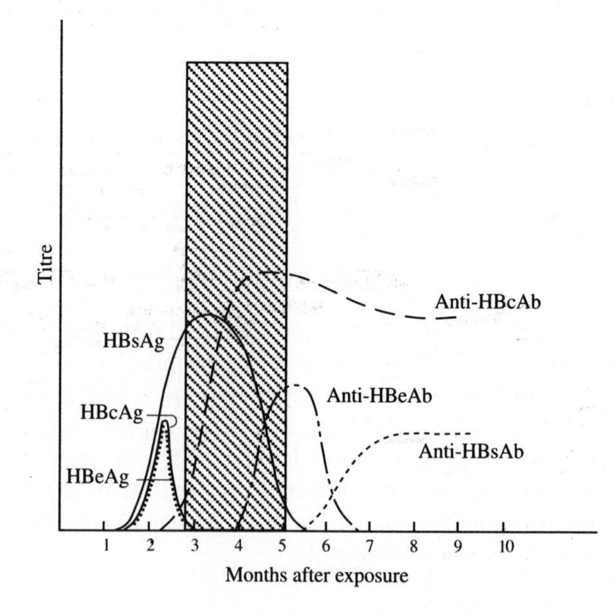

7. D

Seroconversion generally does occur within 3–12 weeks following HIV infection, but one-third to two-thirds of acute infections are associated with an acute mononucleosis-like illness. Acquisition of HIV has been associated with a number of sexually transmitted diseases (STDs), especially ulcerative STDs, for example, syphilis and chancroid. Progression to AIDS is associated with a fall in the CD4/CD8 ratio, but a rise in beta-2-microglobulin (a marker of immune activation). The median time from infection to the development of AIDS is approximately 10 years. The membrane envelope of HIV-1 contains two linked glycoproteins, gp120 and gp41, cleaved from a common precursor, gp160. The nucleocapsid of HIV contains four proteins, p24, p17, p9 and p7, which are cleaved from p53, encoded by the gag gene.

8. A D

L. pneumophila is usually transmitted through environmental water sources (airborne). Diagnosis is made by detecting a significant rise in antibody titre by use of indirect immunofluorescence. Mycoplasma atypical pneumonia causes a rise in cold agglutinins.

9. A C

Viruses which can be vertically acquired include rubella, cytomegalovirus, hepatitis B, HIV, HSV, VZV, enteroviruses and adenovirus. Rubella virus and CMV characteristically cause teratogenic effects (congenital abnormalities), whereas the remaining viruses may cause disseminated infection and disease.

10. A B D

Patients with sickle cell anaemia are at a greatly increased risk of infection with encapsulated organisms, including pneumococci, *Haemophilus influenzae* type b, *Neisseria meningitidis* and *Salmonella enteritides.* In addition to pneumonia, bacteraemia and meningitis, osteomyelitis mainly due to *Salmonella* spp. is a problem in these patients.

11. A C D E

The congenital rubella syndrome includes:

cardiac defects (coarctation of the aorta, patent ductus arteriosus and pulmonary stenosis);
ophthalmic defects (congenital cataracts, retinopathy, glaucoma, choroidoretinitis);

CNS defects (sensorineural deafness, encephalopathy, microencephaly);
endocrine defects (diabetes mellitus, growth retardation, thyroid disease);
reticuloendothelial defects (hepatosplenomegaly, bony lesions on X-ray, thrombocytopenia);
renal defects (polycystic kidneys and renal artery stenosis).

The risk to the fetus is about 90% if the mother has rubella during the first trimester, whereas sensorineural deafness tends to occur if the fetus is affected between 11–16 weeks, after which the risk is very low. Babies with the congenital rubella syndrome excrete virus for long periods – often for more than three months. During this time they are highly infectious. The diagnosis can be made on raised specific IgM titres from cord blood or by direct culture from throat or eye swabs, urine or stool.

12. A B

Specific contraindications to routine vaccination include:

1. Febrile illness, intercurrent infections
2. Hypersensitivity to egg protein contraindicates influenza vaccine; previous anaphylactic reaction to egg contraindicates measles/mumps/rubella, influenza and yellow fever vaccines
3. Infantile eczema

No live vaccine should be administered in:

1. Immunodeficiency or with immunosuppressive therapy, including high-dose corticosteroids
2. Malignancy
3. Pregnancy

13. A D

Toxoplasma gondii is generally asymptomatic in the mother when it is contracted during pregnancy. Toxoplasmosis has widespread effects on the developing brain, causing hydrocephalus, microcephaly, with cerebral calcification and a chorioretinitis. There is usually a resultant mental handicap. If the pregnant woman was infected before conception there is no risk of transmission to the fetus. For maternal toxoplasmosis acquired during pregnancy the risk of congenital toxoplasmosis is 14% during the first trimester, 29% during the second trimester, and 59% during the third trimester (i.e. the risk doubles with each trimester).

14. C D

Escherichia coli is an aerobic, lactose-fermenting non-spore-forming, Gram-negative rod. Although tetracyclines are broadly active against Gram-positive cocci and *E. coli*, many strains, especially those acquired in hospitals, are resistant.

15. A C E

Creutzfeldt–Jakob disease is a slow virus disease with a worldwide prevalence of approximately 1 in 1,000,000. Only 15% of cases are familial and men and women are affected equally. Nosocomial transmission via corneal transplantation has been reported. Brain pathology reveals a spongiform encephalopathy with vacuolation but without inflammation or demyelination.

16. A B C E

Infections acquired from animal sources:

Organism	**Disease or infection**	**Source**
Borrelia burgdorferi	Lyme disease	Birds, deer, mammals
Listeria monocytogenes	Listeriosis	Sheep, cattle
Brucella spp.	Brucellosis	Cattle, sheep, swine, dogs
Toxoplasma gondii	Toxoplasmosis	Cats
Leptospira spp.	Leptospirosis	Dogs, rats, cattle
Yersinia pestis	Plague	Rats
Francisella tularensis	Tularaemia	Deer, rabbits

Humans are the only reservoir for *Salmonella typhi*, the causative agent of typhoid fever. In contrast, many animals may serve as hosts for non-typhoidal *Salmonella* spp.

17. A D E

Exotoxins (extracellular) are produced by most Gram-positive bacteria, e.g. *C. diptheriae, Cl. welchii*, tetanus and botulinum, *B. anthracis*, and *Staph. aureus*, but also a few Gram-negative bacteria, e.g. *V. cholera* and *Shigella*. *E. coli* 0157 is associated with verotoxin-producing strains. The watery diarrhoea associated with *V. cholerae* is due to the action of the enterotoxin.

18. B C D

Bordetella pertussis is only isolated from symptomatic patients. Significant carriage of *Mycobacterium tuberculosis* in the upper respiratory tract in asymptomatic people is uncommon, but small numbers of organisms may lie dormant in healed lesions.

19. A C D E

Toxic epidermal necrolysis is also known as the staphylococcal scalded skin syndrome, and is due to exfoliative toxins (Group II serotype 55 and 71) which cause splitting of desmosomes. Toxic shock syndrome is mediated by the toxic shock syndrome toxin (TSSI) produced by some strains of *Staphylococcus aureus*. Food poisoning is mediated by enterotoxins produced by some strains of *Staphylococcus aureus*.

20. A

Staphylococcus aureus resistant to beta-lactam antibiotics has emerged as an important cause of both community-acquired and nosocomial infections. Beta-lactam resistant isolates are uniformly resistant to methicillin, oxacillin, penicillin and ampicillin. It was previously thought that beta-lactam resistant isolates were less virulent than beta-lactam-susceptible *S. aureus* organisms, however, this is no longer felt to be true. In large hospital outbreaks, spread of beta-lactam-resistant isolates from patient to patient occurs via hospital staff who carry the organism on their hands. Most strains are coagulase positive and catalase negative.

21. A B D

Measles vaccination may be less effective in HIV positive individuals, and consideration should be given to administering normal human immunoglobulins following contact with measles. There have been reports of generalized BCG infection in HIV infected persons. To date, there are insufficient data regarding the safety of yellow fever vaccine in HIV infection.

22. B C

Hepatitis C is a single-stranded RNA virus. The route of infection includes contaminated transfused blood (10%), injecting drug use (40%) and heterosexual contact (10%). The source of infection is unknown in 40%. A serum antibody test has been developed but the actual particle has not been observed nor has it been cultured. Preferred diagnostic tests are multi-antigen EIA anti-HCV: sensitivity is 70–90% in acute HCV, with 80% reactive by 8 weeks. Immunoblot assays are more sensitive and specific. Approximately 80% of patients with transfusion-associated-non-A-non-B hepatitis are anti-HCV positive. HCV may progress to chronic persistent hepatitis, cirrhosis and hepatocellular carcinoma. Chronic hepatitis develops in about half the patients with acute hepatitis C infection. Approximately 10% develop cirrhosis (20% of those with chronic hepatitis). Four studies showed interferon α-2b produced a significant reduction in ALT levels to normal or near normal in 50% of patients, and reduction or elimination of hepatitis C viral RNA from serum. About 50% of responders relapsed within six months of treatment being discontinued.

23. D

There are at least 80 serotypes, many of which cause serious infection. The current vaccine (Pneumovax II) contains 23 serotypes which are most commonly associated with pneumococcal disease. *Streptococcus pneumoniae* may cause acute endocarditis and pericarditis. The *viridans* group of streptococci is responsible for most cases of sub-acute bacterial endocarditis. *Strep. pneumoniae* may become relatively resistant to penicillin, but this resistance is caused by changes in the penicillin-binding proteins of the bacterial cell wall, rather than to production of beta-lactamase. Individuals with sickle cell disease have a 600-fold increase in the risk of serious pneumococcal sepsis. There is evidence to suggest that the full potential for mounting an immunological response to polysaccharide antigens is not reached until about the age of 6 years.

24. A C E

Parvovirus is a DNA virus; specific DNA can be identified by dot-blot hybridization. Approximately 40–60% of the adult population have serological evidence of infection, which is usually acquired between the ages of 4–10 years. Parvovirus B19 has been identified as the cause of erythema infectiosum (Fifth disease) in children. Parvovirus B19 causes aplastic crises in patients with chronic haemolytic anaemia and persistent anaemia from bone marrow depression in immunocompromised individuals.

25. B C D

Helicobacter pylori is a Gram-negative bacterium. It is found in 90% of duodenal ulcers and 70% of gastric ulcer disease, and is found in the mucus of the gastric epithelium as well as in areas of gastric metaplasia in the duodenum. It remains unclear whether eradication of *H. pylori* reduces the relapse rate in gastric ulceration.

26. C D E

Ampicillin and amoxycillin are destroyed by the staphylococcal penicillinase (beta-lactamase). Other effective agents include clindamycin, trimethoprim-sulphamethoxazole and the fluoraquinolones.

27. B D

The enterococci are members of the normal flora of the human gastrointestinal tract. They can also be present in the genitourinary tract, skin and oropharynx. Enterococci can cause a variety of different types of infections. They are a particularly important cause of nosocomial urinary tract infections in patients with indwelling catheters, and of endocarditis in patients with abnormal or prosthetic heart valves. They are frequently isolated with other organisms in intra-abdominal abscesses and in wound infections. Enterococci are less susceptible to penicillins than other streptococci. Enterococci do not cause haemolysis. Species of viridans streptococci include *S. mitior, S. sanguis, S. malleri, S. salivarius* and *S. mutans.*

28. A B C D E

Mechanisms in bacterial food-borne disease:

Preformed toxin	**Toxin production *in vivo***	**Tissue invasion**	**Toxin production and/or tissue invasion**
S. aureus	*C. perfringens*	*C. jejuni*	*V. parahaemolyticus*
B. cereus (short incubation)	*B. cereus*	*Salmonella*	*Y. enterocolitica*
C. botulinum	*C. botulinum*	*Shigella*	
	Enterotoxigenic *E. coli*	Invasive *E. Coli*	
	Verotoxigenic *E. coli*		
	V. cholerae 01 and non-01		

Ciguatera fish poisoning is often characterized by the onset of abdominal cramps, nausea, vomiting and diarrhoea preceded or followed by numbness and parasthesias of the lips, tongue and throat. The illness is caused by ciguatoxin, a poorly characterized lipid soluble compound, which is acquired by fish through the food chain. Ciguatoxin increases membrane sodium permeability and changes the electric potential of cells through its action on sodium channels.

29. A B C D

The most common cause of diarrhoea in travellers is enterotoxigenic *E. coli*, which accounts for one-third to a half of cases. Enteroinvasive *E. coli* and *Shigella* each account for less than 10% of cases of travellers' diarrhoea. The frequency of giardiasis varies widely according to the area visited. Amoebiasis accounts for less than 5% of cases.

30. A B C

Cryptosporidium parvum is spread by contact with infected persons or animals and by contaminated water. It is highly resistant to chlorination. The modified AFB smear of stool samples is now widely used to make the diagnosis. It causes a mild to severe self-limiting disease in healthy persons and life-threatening, relapsing infection in immunocompromised patients. HIV infected individuals are now advised to boil their drinking water. There is no reliable effective therapy.

31. A

Onchocerciasis is treated with ivermectin; *Giardia lamblia* is associated with quinacrine. Itraconazole has some activity against *Aspergillus* spp. The appropriate treatment of toxoplasmosis is sulphadoxine or sulphadiazine in combination with pyrimethamine.

32. B C

True recombination only occurs during meiosis in diploid cells. Transduction refers to transfer of DNA via viruses which infect bacteria (bacteriophages), for example, development of penicillin resistance by *Staph. aureus*. Conjugation refers to mating and direct transfer of DNA (a resistance factor or plasmid) between bacterial cells in contact, for example, development of gentamicin resistance. Mutation refers to changes in the nucleotide sequence of DNA.

33. A

Recombinant hepatitis B vaccine (Recombibax HB or Engerix HB) is a subunit vaccine that contains the surface antigen HBsAg but not the viral core. It is highly effective (approximately 90%) in protecting against hepatitis B infection but offers no cross protection with any other hepatitis virus. There is no increase in side effects when the vaccine is administered to patients who already have antibodies directed against HBsAg. Response rates are lower in persons with HIV infection (50–70%); patients with renal failure (60–70%); diabetes (70–80%) and chronic liver disease (60–70%). The other factors associated with a sub-optimal response to hepatitis B vaccine are obesity, viral 'escape' mutants and older age.

34. A B C D

Chlorhexidine is active mainly against bacteria, but not tubercule bacilli. Chlorhexidine products have limited activity against viruses and none against bacterial spores. Glutaraldehyde is effective against many organisms, including hepatitis B, HIV, and bacterial spores but must only be used when all other alternatives are unsuitable. Hypochlorite is effective against hepatitis B virus, HIV, other viruses and some bacteria.

35. B

Katayama fever (acute schistosomiasis) is acquired by contact with freshwater-harbouring cercarial forms of this parasite. B virus infection is presumed to be acquired through contact with infected Rhesus monkeys. African Rhesus monkeys have recently been reported to have Ebola virus infection. The protozoan, *Leishmania tropica*, is transmitted by the bite of sandflies of the genus *Phlebotomus* and is the cause of the classic 'oriental sore' or cutaneous Leishmaniasis.

36. C D

Dengue fever is predominantly maintained in a human–mosquito–human cycle, though monkeys may also become involved. Yellow fever has two epidemiological patterns: human–mosquito–human, and monkey–mosquito–monkey. Tick-borne encephalitis is transmitted between ticks and rodents, and St Louis encephalitis involves mosquitoes, and birds and pigs.

37. A D

Ganciclovir is phosphorylated by infection-induced kinases. The triphosphate form inhibits viral DNA polymerase. Amantidine inhibits uncoating of virus in the cell through interaction with M_2 protein. The mechanism of action of interferon depends on the virus and cell type, but interferon inhibits:

viral penetration or uncoating;
synthesis of methylation of messenger RNA;
translation of viral proteins;
viral assembly and release.

Stavudine (d4T), as with zidovudine, ddC and ddI, inhibits reverse transcriptase.

1. In cadaveric kidney transplantation

☐ A both CD4 and CD8 cells mediate acute rejection following transplantation
☐ B DRw6-negative grafts have a better outcome than DRw6-positive grafts
☐ C multiple blood transfusions prior to grafting increase the likelihood of graft rejection
☐ D matching for MHC class I antigens is more important than matching for class II antigens in determining graft survival
☐ E the main effect of cyclosporin-A is on CD4 cell-dependent proliferative responses

2. The major histocompatibility complex

☐ A is located on the short arm of chromosome 6
☐ B class II antigens are coded for by A, B and C genes
☐ C class II antigens are more crucial to graft survival than ABO blood group compatibility
☐ D matching at the A and C loci has the greatest influence on graft survival
☐ E non-identical siblings have a 2:4 chance of sharing two antigens

3. The following are examples of antibody-dependent cytotoxic hypersensitivity (type II):

☐ A hyperthyroidism in Graves' disease
☐ B haemolytic anaemia due to *Mycoplasma pneumoniae*
☐ C haemolysis following blood transfusion
☐ D acute early rejection of a transplanted kidney
☐ E hyperacute rejection of a transplanted kidney

4. With regard to cell-mediated (type IV) hypersensitivity

☐ A CD8 cells recognize antigen in conjunction with class I molecules
☐ B this reaction is seen in the acute rejection of a transplanted kidney
☐ C the reaction takes 4–10 hours to develop and persists for several hours
☐ D sensitized T-cells produce lymphokines which attract macrophages
☐ E cell-mediated immunity has been implicated in the protection against some cancers

5. Cell-mediated (type IV/delayed hypersensitivity) reactions are

☐ A dependent on complement
☐ B independent of antibody
☐ C dependent on T-lymphocytes
☐ D usually increased in HIV infected patients
☐ E responsible for autoimmune haemolytic anaemia

6. Major immunological abnormalities in advanced HIV infection include

☐ A marked lymphopenia, especially of cells bearing the CD8 cell marker
☐ B there is a fall in the CD8:CD4 ratio in the peripheral blood
☐ C polyclonal B-cell activation
☐ D increased natural killer cell activity
☐ E impaired delayed cutaneous hypersensitivity response

7. In the HIV-infected individual

☐ A the first antibodies to appear after infection are directed to core proteins
☐ B skin tests to common antigens are usually suppressed
☐ C cyclosporin-A inhibits the reverse transcriptase enzyme of the virus
☐ D soluble CD4 molecules bind to HIV and block its infectivity
☐ E the diagnosis is usually confirmed by positive isolation and culture of HIV

8. Rheumatoid factor

- ☐ A is usually IgM
- ☐ B is directed against the Fc fragment of the patient's own IgM
- ☐ C is present in high titre in 70% of patients with rheumatoid arthritis
- ☐ D must be present for the diagnosis of rheumatoid arthritis
- ☐ E is found in 50% of SLE patients

9. Complement levels are abnormal in

- ☐ A minimal change glomerulonephritis
- ☐ B SLE
- ☐ C ataxia telangiectasia
- ☐ D hereditary angioneurotic oedema
- ☐ E mesangiocapillary glomerulonephritis

10. The following statements are true:

- ☐ A B lymphocytes are characterized by rosette formation when mixed with sheep red cells
- ☐ B IgG and IgE are the only antibodies which are small enough to cross the placenta
- ☐ C rheumatoid factor is an acute phase protein
- ☐ D B lymphocytes make up 70% of blood lymphocytes
- ☐ E IgE represents up to 10% of the total immunoglobulins in the serum

11. Hypogammaglobulinaemia occurs in the following conditions:

- ☐ A kala-azar
- ☐ B SLE
- ☐ C multiple sclerosis
- ☐ D nephrotic syndrome
- ☐ E polymyositis

12. Antinuclear antibodies (ANA) are usually absent in

☐ A dermatomyositis
☐ B polyarteritis nodosa
☐ C rheumatoid arthritis
☐ D infective endocarditis
☐ E scleroderma

13. Soluble circulating immune complexes may be found in

☐ A myasthenia gravis
☐ B infective endocarditis
☐ C Rhesus haemolytic disease
☐ D dermatitis herpetiformis
☐ E post-streptococcal glomerulonephritis

14. Delayed hypersensitivity is depressed in

☐ A Hodgkin's disease
☐ B scleroderma
☐ C sarcoidosis
☐ D malnutrition
☐ E Wiscott–Aldrich syndrome

15. Tumour necrosis factor

☐ A is produced in the necrotic centre of tumours
☐ B is a cytokine produced by monocytes
☐ C causes toxic shock syndrome
☐ D is the predominant cause of shock in Gram-negative septicaemia
☐ E increases capillary permeability

16. BCG should be given to the following:

- ☐ A a 13-year-old HIV positive child
- ☐ B a 7-year-old immigrant child from Bangladesh
- ☐ C an unvaccinated Mantoux negative adult contact of a person with active pulmonary tuberculosis
- ☐ D an adult immigrant from Bangladesh
- ☐ E Mantoux positive schoolchildren

17. IgA

- ☐ A has a key role in mucosal immunity
- ☐ B has four distinct subgroups
- ☐ C activates complement via the classical pathway
- ☐ D is manufactured in the lymph nodes
- ☐ E crosses the placenta

18. Leukotrienes

- ☐ A increase vascular permeability
- ☐ B include the slow-reacting substance of anaphylaxis (SRS-A)
- ☐ C cause bronchodilation
- ☐ D mast cells are an important source
- ☐ E are derived from palmitic acid

19. The acute phase response

- ☐ A is stimulated by cytokines
- ☐ B may occur post-operatively
- ☐ C may be assessed by measurement of C-peptide
- ☐ D is particularly marked with viral infections
- ☐ E causes a reduction in plasma viscosity

20. The following are associated with the presence of cytoplasmic anti-neutrophil cytoplasmic antibodies (ANCA):

☐ A systemic lupus erythematosus
☐ B Wegener's granulomatosis
☐ C rheumatoid arthritis
☐ D microscopic polyarteritis
☐ E scleroderma

21. Treatment with intravenous immunoglobulin is appropriate in the following conditions:

☐ A chronic lymphocytic leukaemia
☐ B nephrotic syndrome
☐ C X-linked hypogammaglobulinaemia
☐ D the acquired immunodeficiency syndrome in a child
☐ E isolated IgA deficiency

22. Immunoglobulin M

☐ A is predominantly extravascular
☐ B has 8 antigen binding sites
☐ C concentration is increased in the serum of patients with untreated coeliac disease
☐ D is responsible for the determination of blood group
☐ E is the main component of rheumatoid factor

23. The following conditions occur more commonly in patients with Bruton's congenital agammaglobulinaemia:

☐ A sinusitis
☐ B pneumonia
☐ C chronic meningoencephalitis due to echovirus
☐ D life-threatening measles
☐ E chronic lymphatic leukaemia

24. The following cytokines are correctly paired with the appropriate actions:

- ☐ A interleukin-1 – enhances PMN adherence and bactericidal activity
- ☐ B interleukin-1 – direct antiviral and antitumour activity
- ☐ C tumour necrosis factor – induces catabolic state and fever
- ☐ D interleukin-γ and interleukin-2 – inflammatory mediators
- ☐ E granulocyte/macrophage colony stimulating factor – inhibition of granulocyte precursors

25. The following skin conditions are matched with the correct finding on direct immunofluorescent examination of a skin biopsy:

- ☐ A pemphigoid – autoantibodies to basement membrane zone
- ☐ B pemphigus – granular deposits of IgA in dermal papilla
- ☐ C dermatitis herpetiformis – autoantibodies to epidermal intercellular cement
- ☐ D SLE – deposits of immunoglobulin and complement along basement membrane zone
- ☐ E SLE – deposits of immunoglobulins at the dermal–epidermal junction of unaffected skin in the lupus band test

26. The following features are characteristic of the primary antiphospholipid syndrome:

- ☐ A antibodies to double-stranded DNA are present in more than 60% of patients
- ☐ B deep vein thrombosis is the commonest presentation
- ☐ C lupus anticoagulant is a more frequent finding than in SLE
- ☐ D in common with SLE, the prolonged clotting time corrects with normal plasma
- ☐ E the ratio of female to male cases is 2:1

27. The following micro-organisms use antigenic variation as a major means of evading host defences:

☐ A *Streptococcus pneumoniae*
☐ B *Mycobacterium tuberculosis*
☐ C Influenza A virus
☐ D *Neisseria meningitidis*
☐ E *Trypanosoma brucei*

28. Which of the following statements about interferon-alfa are true:

☐ A it is useful in the treatment of chronic hepatitis B infection
☐ B it induces differentiation of natural killer cells
☐ C it suppresses natural killer cell activity
☐ D genetically engineered recombinant interferon is available
☐ E it is therapeutically useful in hairy cell leukaemia

29. Features characteristic of a type I T-helper cell response (TH_1) include

☐ A IL-2 secretion
☐ B production of IgE
☐ C development of a granuloma
☐ D a cell-mediated immune response
☐ E interferon-γ production

30. Antimitochondrial antibodies are

☐ A found in about 50% of patients with primary biliary cirrhosis
☐ B found in 20% of patients with SLE
☐ C responsible for the bile duct damage seen in primary biliary cirrhosis
☐ D associated with the presence of the HLA-$A1_1$, -$B8_1$, -DR3 haplotype
☐ E accompanied frequently by a rise in IgM antibodies in patients with chronic active hepatitis

31. The following statements about the MHC are correct:

- ☐ A class II MHC region products are expressed on almost all nucleated cells
- ☐ B the MHC is remarkable for its extreme degree of polymorphism
- ☐ C the CD4 molecule interacts with the non-polymorphic region of the class II molecule
- ☐ D cytotoxic T-cells recognize antigen alongside class I molecules
- ☐ E antigens are usually processed before being presented to T-cells by the MHC

32. The following cells are known to be involved in the initial presentation of antigen to T-cells:

- ☐ A macrophages
- ☐ B neutrophils
- ☐ C follicular dendritic cells
- ☐ D $CD8^{+}$ cells
- ☐ E red cells

ANSWERS AND TEACHING NOTES: IMMUNOLOGY

1. A E

DRw6-positivity and multiple blood transfusions (before surgery) have a beneficial effect on outcome following renal transplantation. However, the benefit of previous transfusions on graft survival is now probably marginal with better tissue typing and the use of cyclosporin A. In renal transplantation, matching for MHC class II antigens is more important than matching for class I antigens in determining graft survival. Cyclosporin A prevents the activation of T-lymphocytes by inhibiting signal transduction within the cytoplasm of T-cells. Its major effect is inhibition of interleukin-2 (IL-2) production and thus $CD4^+$ cell-dependent proliferative responses. NK cell activity is also affected since it is dependent on IL-2 activity. It reduces the incidence of organ rejection and graft versus host (GVH) disease.

2. A E

Class I HLA-antigens are coded for by A, B and C genes, which are present on all nucleated cells and determine graft rejection. Class II antigens are coded for by DP, DQ and DR genes and are present on monocytes/macrophages, B-lymphocytes and occasionally activated T-lymphocytes. ABO compatibility (not identical) is essential for transplant viability. The HLA-DR locus is the most important locus governing graft rejection. Non-identical siblings have a 1:4 chance of sharing all four HLA antigens and 1:4 chance of having no antigens in common.

3. B C E

In cell bound hypersensitivity (type II), circulating antibody (IgG or IgM) binds to cell-membrane receptors and activates complement which, in turn, mediates lysis and phagocytosis. Graves' disease is an example of type V hypersensitivity (stimulatory) where IgG antibodies (long acting thyroid stimulator, LATS) results in prolonged secretion of thyroid hormone. Acute early rejection and GVH disease are examples of cell-mediated hypersensitivity (type IV). Hyperacute rejection is due to pre-formed circulating cytotoxic antibody which reacts with MHC class I antigens in the donor organ. (See the table accompanying the answer to Question 5.)

4. B D E

Type IV reactions are initiated by T-cells which react with antigen and release lymphokines. These, in turn, attract other cells, especially macrophages. Type IV hypersensitivity usually starts hours or days after contact with the antigen and persists for days. The CD8 cells recognize antigen in conjunction with MHC class II molecules. Other clinically important examples include contact dermatitis and the tuberculin skin reaction.

5. **B C**

Type IV hypersensitivity reactions depend on T-lymphocytes, but are independent of antibodies and complement. They are usually decreased in HIV infection where there is depletion of CD4 cells. Autoimmune haemolytic anaemia is an example of a type II reaction. Type II (cell-bound) and Type III (immune complex) hypersensitivity are mediated by complement.

	Mechanism	**Hypersensitivity Consequences**	**Disease**
Type I (immediate)	IgE Mast cells Basophils IgG_4	Vasodilatation Eosinophils attracted Histamine Leukotrienes, etc.	Atopic diseases, e.g. asthma
Type II (cell-bound antigen)	IgM IgG	Complement activation Cell lysis Opsonization Neutrophil activation Cell stimulation Blocking Ab	Autoimmune haemolytic anaemia Myasthenia gravis Idiopathic thrombocytopenic purpura Goodpasture's syndrome Graves' disease Pernicious anaemia
Type III (immune complex)	IgG IgA	Circulating immune complexes Complement activation	Serum sickness SLE Henoch–Schonlein Vasculitides Glomerulonephritis
Type IV (delayed)	T-cells Macrophages/ Antigen-presenting cells	Attraction and activation of lymphocytes and moncytes	Tuberculosis Graft rejection Graft versus host disease Rheumatoid arthritis

6. C E

The most striking effects of HIV are on T-cell-mediated responses, with a fall in the absolute number of CD4⁺ T-cells and in the CD4:CD8 ratios. There is an associated rise in the number of CD8 suppressor/cytotoxic cells. As the disease progresses, patients show anergy in their delayed-hypersensitivity skin test, such as the tuberculin test. There is decreased natural killer cell function.

7. B D

The first antibodies to appear, following HIV infection, are directed against the envelope glycoproteins (gp120 and gp41) and appear usually 3 weeks to 3 months after exposure. The diagnosis of HIV infection is usually confirmed by finding HIV-antibody in serum (ELISA technique). If the ELISA test is positive then a Western blot is usually performed. Combining these two tests, the false positive rate is 1 in 140,000. The principal action of cyclosporin is to suppress lymphokine production by T-helper cells, by interfering with the activation of lymphokine genes.

8. A C

Rheumatoid factor can be IgM, IgG or IgA. It is directed against the Fc segment of IgG. It is found in 20–30% of SLE patients. Approximately 70% of patients with aggressive rheumatoid disease have rheumatoid factor in their serum (seropositive RA), whereas a subgroup with moderate disease lacks circulatory rheumatoid factor (seronegative RA).

9. B D E

Low complement levels occur in certain diseases and many correlate with disease activity, for example in post-streptococcal glomerulonephritis, SLE nephritis, infectious endocarditis, membranoproliferative glomerulonephritis, serum sickness, liver disease, septicaemia and disseminated intravascular coagulation. Inherited C1 inhibitor deficiency is associated with hereditary angioneurotic oedema (due to uncontrolled complement activation).

10. None correct

B-cells are identified by cell-surface immunoglobin receptors; T-cells are identified by rosette formation with sheep red blood cells and comprise 70–80% of blood lymphocyte population. IgG is the only immunoglobulin that crosses the placenta. IgE represents approximately 0.002% of total immunoglobulin levels in the serum.

11. A B D E

Severe hypogammaglobulinaemia can occur as a secondary phenomenon in a number of other diseases, e.g. protein-losing enteropathy (classically seen in intestinal lymphangiectasia), myelomatosis, chronic lymphocytic leukaemia and congenital rubella.

12. A B

Antinuclear antibodies (ANAs) are IgG or IgM antibodies directed against a variety of nuclear constituents, e.g. DNA or RNA. High titres occur in SLE, other connective tissue disorders (e.g. Sjogren's syndrome, systemic sclerosis, rheumatoid arthritis), autoimmune diseases (e.g. chronic active hepatitis, myasthenia gravis), and with the use of certain drugs, e.g. drug-induced SLE syndrome. There are four patterns of nuclear staining for ANAs.

Pattern	Disease association	Antigen
Homogeneous	Common pattern	DNA histone
Speckled	SLE, Sjogren's syndrome, mixed connective tissue disorder	Extractable nuclear antigen
Nucleolar	Scleroderma, SLE	Nucleolar DNA
Centromere	CREST syndrome, diffuse scleroderma	Centromere

13. B E

Three different mechanisms are responsible for diseases resulting from immune-complex formation:

1. The combined effects of a low grade persistent infection (e.g. alpha-haemolytic *Streptococcus viridans*, *Plasmodium vivax*, or viral hepatitis), together with a weak antibody response.
2. A complication of autoimmune disease where the continued production of antibody to a self-antigen leads to prolonged immune-complex formation, e.g. rheumatoid arthritis, SLE, polyarteritis, polymyositis/dermatomyositis, cutaneous vasculitis, fibrosing alveolitis and cryoglobulinaemia.

3. Formation of immune complexes at body surfaces, notably in the lungs, following repeated inhalation of antigenic materials from moulds, plants or animals, e.g. Farmer's lung and Pigeon Fancier's lung.

14. A C D E

Delayed hypersensitivity reactions are impaired in patients with sarcoidosis, malignant lymphomas, the di George syndrome and those receiving corticosteroid therapy. Impaired delayed hypersensitivity increases susceptibility to opportunistic infections (e.g. fungi and *Pneumocystis carinii*) and severe viral infections. Immunization with live vaccines may cause fatal generalized reactions. The Wiskott–Aldrich syndrome is a combined B- and T-cell disorder with an X-linked inheritance.

15. B D E

Tumour necrosis factor (TNF) is a cytokine released by the macrophages/monocytes. It is the principal mediator of the host response to Gram-negative bacteria, but may also play a role in the response to other infectious organisms. It activates inflammatory leucocytes to kill microbes, stimulates mononuclear phagocytes to produce cytokines, acts as a co-stimulator for T-cell activation and antibody production by B-cells, and exerts an interferon-like effect against viruses. It enhances the microbicidal capacity of macrophages and neutrophils, causes NK cells to release interferon-γ, and causes changes in endothelial cells increasing the entry of cells into sites of inflammation.

16. B C D

Previously unvaccinated Mantoux-negative health workers or contacts of persons with active pulmonary tuberculosis should receive BCG. Other indications include neonates born in households where there is active TB, immigrants from countries with a high prevalence of TB and their children, wherever born. BCG is contraindicated in immunosuppressed patients.

17. A C

IgA is the principal immunoglobulin in secretions of the respiratory and gastrointestinal tract, and in sweat, saliva, tears and colostrum. IgA has a key defence role for mucosal surfaces. It polymerises to a dimer intracellularly by binding through a cysteine-rich polypeptide JC chain synthesized locally by mucosal cells. When aggregated, it binds polymorphs and activates complement by the alternative pathway.

18. A B D

The leukotrienes are synthesized by leucocytes and mast cells and are mediators of inflammation and allergic reactions. They produce arteriolar constriction and bronchoconstriction, increase vascular permeability and attract neutrophils and eosinophils to inflammatory sites. Leukotriene D4 has been identified as SRS-A which causes smooth muscle contraction. Prostaglandins, prostacyclins, thromboxanes and leucotrienes are derived from arachodonic acid via the cycloxygenase and lipoxygenase pathway.

19. A B

The acute phase proteins include proteins which act as mediators (as in opsonization-C3 and C4 complement components, C-reactive protein), enzyme inhibitors (α_1-antitrypsin) or scavengers (haptoglobin). Inflammation activates macrophages and lymphocytes to produce cytokines (particularly interleukin 6), which stimulate the production of acute phase proteins from the liver. C-reactive protein is used to measure the acute phase response. C-peptide is produced in the pancreas during the manufacture of insulin. There is only a minor acute phase response in viral (compared with bacterial) infections. An acute phase response may occur in inflammatory conditions, after trauma, post-operatively, associated with malignancy and in autoimmune disease.

20. B D

Antineutrophil cytoplasmic antibodies (ANCA) are present in more than 95% of patients with active generalized Wegener's granulomatosis. They are found frequently in patients with various forms of vasculitis with or without renal impairment, but rarely in patients with immune-complex nephritis. ANCA-associated glomerulonephritis is now the most commonly recognized form of rapidly progressive glomerulonephritis.

21. A C D

In nephrotic syndrome, although IgG levels may be low, IgG antibody formation is normal. Unlike adults with AIDS, children have not had the opportunity to develop antibodies to a wide variety of antigens before the onset of their defective immune response and therefore intravenous immunoglobulin may have a role in their management. In isolated IgA deficiency, where total IgG levels are normal or elevated, intravenous immunoglobulin treatment is contraindicated. Such patients may have IgA antibodies resulting in anaphylactic shock if the administered gamma globulin contains IgA. There is no effective replacement therapy for IgA currently available.

22. D E

IgM antibody is a macroglobulin made up of five monomeric immunoglobulin subunits. It is mainly intravascular. It activates complement via the classical pathway and is unable to cross the placenta. It is the principal immunoglobulin of the primary immune response. The presence of high levels of specific fetal IgM indicates intrauterine infection, e.g. rubella. IgM has a half-life of approximately 5 days. The serum concentration of IgM is characteristically reduced in patients with untreated coeliac disease and may increase to normal with a gluten-free diet. Blood group antibodies are of the IgM type. Rheumatoid factors are IgM antibodies to IgG.

23. A B C

Bruton's agammaglobulinaemia is a rare X-linked inherited disorder that presents in male infants at about 6 months with recurrent pyogenic and gastrointestinal infections. Circulating B-cells are absent, but T-cells are normal or increased. Infections with *Staphylococcus*, *Streptococcus* and *Haemophilus* are common, but these patients are also susceptible to enteroviruses, e.g. echoviruses. Recurrent sinopulmonary infections are characteristic. The defective gene (tyrosine-kinase mutation) on the X chromosome has been identified.

24. A C D

Both interleukin-1 (IL-1) and tumour necrosis factor (TNF) increase endothelial adherence and procoagulant activities, and induce a catabolic state and fever. Only tumour necrosis factor has direct antiviral and anti-tumour activity. Cytokines, IL-2, IFN-γ and TNF are inflammatory mediators produced by T-helper type I (TH_1) cells. Granulocyte/macrophage colony-stimulating factor is responsible for the growth and differentiation of macrophage and monocyte precursors.

25. A D

Pemphigus is associated with autoantibodies to epidermal intracellular cement, and dermatitis herpetiformis with coarse granular deposits of IgA in dermal papilla. In bullous skin eruptions, direct immunofluorescence of perilesional skin rather than established bullae is diagnostic.

26. B C E

Patients with high titre antiphospholipid antibodies (primary antiphospholipid antibody syndrome) are at a greatly increased risk of recurrent fetal loss and recurrent thrombosis (arterial or venous). The frequency of different presentations is as follows:

deep vein thrombosis	54%
arterial thrombosis	44%
recurrent fetal loss	34%
pulmonary embolism	18%
cerebrovascular accident	13%

Such patients should be anticoagulated for life. There is considerable overlap in the clinical features associated with both antiphospholipid antibodies and lupus anticoagulant. In common with both SLE and the APA syndrome, the clotting defect fails to correct with normal plasma, implying that an antibody is present. The syndrome is associated with a false positive VDRL.

Comparison of SLE with primary antiphospholipid (APA) syndrome

	SLE	**APA syndrome**
Female:Male	9:1	2:1
Mean age (years)	24	38
Antinuclear antibody (%)	>90	45
Antibodies to double-stranded DNA (%)	80	0
Lupus anticoagulant (%)	10	60
Antiphospholipid antibodies (%)	40	100

27. C D E

Antigenic variation is best recognized in trypanosomiasis and influenza but also in some bacteria, such as meningococci. After infection with *Trypanosoma brucei,* destruction of trypanosomes by host antibody is followed by emergence of parasites expressing different surface antigens, or variant surface glucoproteins. This type of antigenic variation is known as phenotypic variation, in contrast to genotypic variation, in which a new strain periodically results in an epidemic, e.g. influenza virus.

28. A B D E

Interferon-alpha (IFN-α) is released by monocytes and has an anti-viral action by activation of natural killer cells, upregulation of MHC class I antigens on virally infected cells and inhibition of viral replication. Genetically engineered recombinant IFN-α, β and γ are available but interferon-α is the best studied. IFN-α has a role in the management of poorly responsive malignancies, such as hairy cell leukaemia and renal cell carcinoma, and also acts as an antiviral agent, producing significant clearing of hepatitis B in chronic carriers, and histological improvement in 50% of patients with hepatitis C.

29. A C D E

Recent work has shown that $CD4^+$ T-cells can be divided into different subsets depending on their cytokine profile. CD4 cells that produce IL-2 and IFN-γ but not IL-4 are designated TH_1 and are chiefly responsible for delayed type hypersensitivity responses. In contrast, CD4 T-cells that produce IL-4 and IL-5, but not IL-2 or IFN-γ are designated TH_2. They are efficient helper cells for antibody production, especially IgE and IgG_1.

30. None correct

Over 95% of patients with primary biliary cirrhosis (PBC) have circulating antimitochondrial antibodies; the absence of these antibodies virtually excludes the diagnosis. Mitochondrial antibodies are also found in a small proportion of patients with chronic active hepatitis (CAH) or cirrhosis of unknown aetiology. The cause of the bile duct damage in PBC is unclear but may be mediated by cytotoxic T-cells. Unlike CAH, PBC is not associated with any particular HLA antigens. IgM is raised in >80% of patients with PBC; IgG is elevated in CAH.

31. B C D E

Class II MHC molecules have a restricted distribution compared to class I molecules which are found in most tissues. Class II molecules are normally found on B-lymphocytes, activated T-cells, macrophages and inflamed vascular endothelium. Human histocompatibility antigens are remarkable for their degree of polymorphism, i.e. the genetic variability between individuals is very great and most unrelated individuals possess different HLA molecules. Antigen processing is crucial for the recognition of antigen by T-cells. Processed antigen is presented to T-cells alongside the MHC class II antigens on the surface of specialized cells – known as antigen-presenting cells (APCs). T-cells do not recognize processed antigen alone. CD4 helper T-cells recognize antigen with class II molecules, and CD8 suppressor/cytotoxic T-cells recognize antigens with MHC class I molecules.

32. A C

Antigen presenting cells (APCs) are a heterogeneous population of leucocytes that are found primarily in the skin, lymph nodes, spleen and thymus. They may have a pivotal role in the induction of the functional activity of T-helper cells, or communicate with other leucocytes. The classic APCs are the Langerhans cells in the skin, and the follicular dendriditic cells, found in the secondary follicles of the B-cell areas of the lymph nodes and spleen. The Langerhans cells are rich in class II MHC for communicating with CD4 and T-cells, whereas follicular dendritic cells do not express class II MHC. B-cells and macrophages are also efficient as antigen-presenting cells.

5: ANATOMY

1. The subclavian artery

☐ A has a surface marking indicated by an arch between the sterno-clavicular joint and mid-clavicle
☐ B passes superficial to the scalenus anterior
☐ C gives off the thyrocervical trunk
☐ D arises from the brachiocephalic trunk on the left side
☐ E gives off the vertebral artery

2. The following reflexes and innervating spinal segments are correctly paired:

☐ A ankle jerk – S1
☐ B knee jerk – L3 and L4
☐ C biceps jerk – C7 and C8
☐ D triceps jerk – T1
☐ E anal reflex – S1

3. The left principal bronchus

☐ A runs more vertically than the right bronchus
☐ B is longer than the right bronchus
☐ C divides into 10 tertiary bronchi
☐ D contains complete cartilaginous rings
☐ E divides into three secondary bronchi

4. A complete division of the femoral nerve results in

☐ A foot drop
☐ B paraesthesia of the lateral aspect of the foot
☐ C failure of knee extension
☐ D sensory loss over the medial part of the lower leg
☐ E failure of adduction of the thigh at the hip joint

5. An injury to the ulnar nerve at the wrist results in

☐ A wasting of the thenar eminence
☐ B claw hand
☐ C loss of the pincer-like action of the thumb and index finger
☐ D sensory impairment over the palmar surface of the medial one and a half fingers
☐ E wasting of the 2nd lumbrical muscle

6. The abdominal aorta

☐ A pierces the diaphragm in front of the T12 vertebra
☐ B divides into the two common iliac arteries in front of L4
☐ C gives off five lumbar arteries on each side
☐ D is closely related to the left sympathetic trunk
☐ E aneurysms usually arise above the origin of the renal arteries

7. The thoracic duct

☐ A enters the thorax through the caval opening of the diaphragm
☐ B bends laterally in front of the carotid sheath at the level of C7 vertebra
☐ C passes anterior to the left phrenic nerve at the medial border of the scalenus anterior muscle
☐ D passes behind the first part of the subclavian artery
☐ E terminates in the left internal jugular vein

8. The median nerve

☐ A derives its fibres from spinal segments C6–8 and T1
☐ B gives off a muscular branch to the triceps
☐ C supplies the ulnar half of the flexor digitorum profundus
☐ D damage at the wrist causes wasting of the hypothenar muscles
☐ E gives off sensory branches to the dorsal aspects of the lateral two and a half fingers

9. The following muscles and nerves supplying them are correctly matched:

- ☐ A chief supinator of the forearm – deep branch of the radial nerve (C7, 8)
- ☐ B extensors of the hand at the wrist joint – deep branch of the radial nerve (C7)
- ☐ C quadriceps – femoral nerve (L3, 4)
- ☐ D opposition of thumb and fingers – median nerve (C8)
- ☐ E ankle dorsiflexion – sciatic (tibial) nerve (S1, 2)

10. The following cutaneous areas and sensory roots are correctly paired:

- ☐ A the sole of the foot – S3
- ☐ B the little finger – T1
- ☐ C the groin – L5
- ☐ D the umbilicus – T10
- ☐ E the index finger – C5

11. The following statements about the spinal cord are correct:

- ☐ A the subdural space contains the cerebrospinal fluid (CSF)
- ☐ B segment T12 lies at the level of vertebral body T11
- ☐ C it transmits two-point discrimination sensations in the lateral spinothalamic tract
- ☐ D hemisection results in contralateral upper motor neuron paralysis below the level of the lesion
- ☐ E hemisection results in contralateral loss of pain and temperature sensation below the level of the lesion

12. Porto-systemic anastomoses occur in the following sites:

- ☐ A around the umbilicus
- ☐ B the middle third of the oesophagus
- ☐ C the lower end of the rectum
- ☐ D the bare area of the liver
- ☐ E the appendix

13. The clinical features of an injury to the common peroneal nerve include

- ☐ A a claw-like deformity of the toes
- ☐ B positive Trendelenburg test
- ☐ C sensation lost in the sole of the foot
- ☐ D equinovarus deformity of the foot
- ☐ E calcaneovalgus deformity of the foot

14. The facial nerve

- ☐ A gives off the chorda tympani nerve 5 mm below the stylomastoid foramen
- ☐ B if the intracranial part of the nerve is involved, there is loss of taste over the anterior two-thirds of the tongue
- ☐ C if the intracranial part of the nerve is involved, the stapedius reflex is preserved
- ☐ D supplies secretomotor fibres to the submandibular gland
- ☐ E if injured at a supranuclear level, the forehead muscles are paralysed

15. The clinical features of a lumbar disc prolapse affecting the S1 root only include

- ☐ A paraesthesia on the medial aspect of the foot
- ☐ B a positive femoral stretch test
- ☐ C weakness and wasting of the dorsiflexors of the foot
- ☐ D limitation of straight leg raising
- ☐ E impaired knee jerk

16. The oesophagus

- ☐ A is crossed by the left main bronchus
- ☐ B is a site for a portal–systemic anastomosis at its lower third
- ☐ C lies in front of part of the descending aorta
- ☐ D extends from the level of C6 to the level of the 6th thoracic vertebra
- ☐ E the lower third is the commonest site for carcinoma of the oesophagus

17. The radial nerve

☐ A derives its fibres from segments C6–8 and T1 of the brachial plexus
☐ B gives off a muscular branch to biceps
☐ C gives off sensory branches to the dorsal aspect of the radial half to the hand
☐ D injury at the elbow results in loss of pronation of the forearm
☐ E supplies the triceps muscle

18. The internal jugular vein

☐ A begins at the jugular foramen as a continuation of the sigmoid sinus
☐ B passes behind the thoracic duct on the left side
☐ C runs alongside a chain of deep cervical lymph nodes
☐ D lies medial to the internal carotid artery within the carotid sheath
☐ E joins the subclavian vein to form the brachiocephalic vein

19. With respect to development of the thyroid gland

☐ A follicular cells arise from the epithelium of the dorsal wing of the fourth pharyngeal pouch
☐ B parafollicular cells arise from the fifth pharyngeal pouch
☐ C approximately 50% of thyroglossal cysts lie close to or just inferior to the body of the hyoid bone
☐ D thyroglossal cysts may lie at the base of the tongue
☐ E a thyroglossal fistula usually arises due to rupture of a thyroglossal cyst

20. The inferior vena cava (IVC)

☐ A is formed by the two common iliac veins anterior to the right common iliac artery
☐ B pierces the diaphragm at the level of the T12 vertebra
☐ C directly receives the left suprarenal vein
☐ D runs to the right of the aorta
☐ E receives the two hepatic veins

21. Injury to the T1 root of the brachial plexus may result in

☐ A an Erb–Duchenne paralysis
☐ B loss of elbow flexion
☐ C loss of cutaneous sensation over the anterior surface of the palm and fingers
☐ D a 'claw hand'
☐ E Horner's syndrome

22. The following muscles assist in the inversion of the foot:

☐ A tibialis anterior
☐ B tibialis posterior
☐ C peroneus longus
☐ D all tendons of extensor digitorum longus
☐ E flexor hallucis longus

23. Lesions at the following sites of the visual system and the resulting visual field deficit are correctly paired:

☐ A the optic chiasma – bitemporal hemianopia
☐ B the optic tract – ipsilateral homonymous hemianopia
☐ C the optic radiation in the temporal lobe – contralateral inferior homonymous quadrantanopia
☐ D the optic radiation in the parietal lobe – contralateral superior homonymous quadrantanopia
☐ E the visual cortex – contralateral homonymous hemianopia with macular sparing

24. The following areas of the central nervous system and the main supplying arteries are correctly paired:

☐ A Broca's area – the anterior cerebral artery
☐ B Wernicke's area – the middle cerebral artery
☐ C the visual cortex – the posterior cerebral artery
☐ D the anterior two-thirds of the spinal cord – branches of the posterior inferior cerebellar arteries
☐ E the auditory cortex – the middle cerebral artery

25. If the corticospinal pathway is injured on the left side at the C2 cord level you would expect to find

- ☐ A weakness of limb muscles – on the left side
- ☐ B brisk reflexes – on the left side
- ☐ C spasticity of muscles – on the left side
- ☐ D spasticity of muscles – on the right side
- ☐ E upgoing plantar – on the right side

26. A left homonymous hemianopia can be produced by a lesion in the right

- ☐ A occipital cortex
- ☐ B optic radiation
- ☐ C optic tract
- ☐ D optic nerve
- ☐ E Edinger–Westphal nucleus

27. Complete transection of the thoracic cord is characterized by

- ☐ A permanent loss of voluntary control of lower limb muscles
- ☐ B permanent loss of tendon reflexes in the lower limb
- ☐ C permanent loss of sensation below the level of the lesion
- ☐ D return of voluntary sphincteric function
- ☐ E impotence

1. **A C E**

   The subclavian artery originates on the right from the brachiocephalic trunk, and on the left from the aortic arch. It passes deep to the scalenus anterior muscle and becomes the axillary artery at the lateral border of the 1st rib. Its branches include the vertebral, the internal thoracic, deep cervical and highest intercostal arteries and the thyrocervical trunk.

2. **A B**

   The tibial branch of the sciatic nerve mediates the ankle jerk and the femoral nerve mediates the knee jerk. The biceps jerk is mediated by the musculocutaneous nerve (C5 and C6). The innervating segments for the triceps jerk and anal reflex are C7 and S3 and S4, respectively.

3. **B C**

   The right bronchus is wider, shorter (2.5 cm) and more vertical than the left (5 cm), therefore foreign bodies are more likely to enter the right bronchus. The left bronchus divides into two secondary bronchi and 10 tertiary ones (there are 10 bronchopulmonary segments). The right bronchus divides into three secondary bronchi and 10 tertiary ones. The main bronchi contain C-shaped cartilaginous rings.

4. **C D**

   The femoral nerve supplies the muscles of the anterolateral thigh, the quadriceps (knee extension) and the sartorius muscles. The sensory branches innervate the anteromedial thigh and the medial aspect of the lower leg and foot (the saphenous branch). Footdrop and paraesthesia over the lateral aspect of the foot result from damage to the common peroneal nerve. Hip adduction muscles are mainly supplied by the obturator nerve.

5. **B D**

   With ulnar nerve damage at the wrist, there is wasting and paralysis of the hypothenar muscles, and intrinsic hand muscles (apart from the lateral two lumbricals), resulting in a 'claw hand'. The clawing is less marked if the injury occurs at the elbow level due to additional paralysis of flexor digitorum profundus. The median nerve innervates the muscles of the thenar eminence (opponens pollicis, abductor pollicis, and flexor pollicis brevis) and the 1st and 2nd lumbricals.

   LOAF

The distribution of the loss of sensation is shown below.

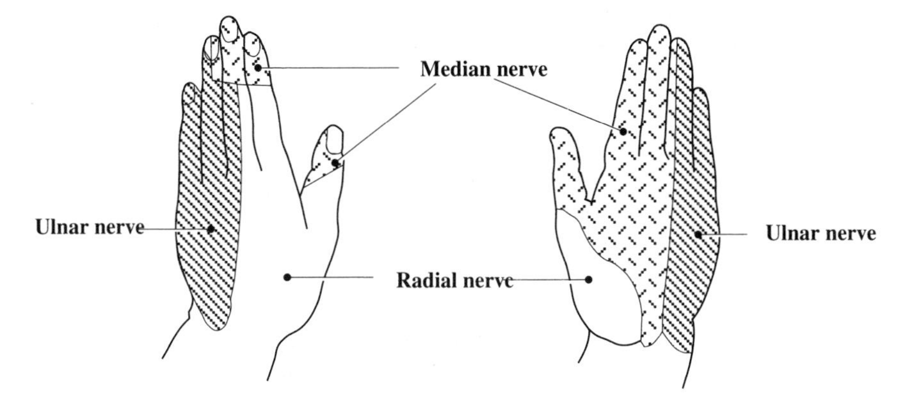

6. A B D

The branches of the abdominal aorta include: suprarenal, renal, gonadal, coeliac, superior mesenteric, inferior mesenteric, inferior phrenic, four lumbar, median sacral, left and right common iliac arteries. Aortic aneurysms are usually atherosclerotic in origin and lie infrarenally in 95% of cases. The abdominal aorta lies on the vertebral column and its ligaments, and the inferior vena cava to the right of it.

7. C E

The thoracic duct drains the whole lymphatic field below the diaphragm and the left half of the lymphatics above it. It begins at and passes superiorly from the cisterna chyli to enter the thorax through the aortic opening on the right side of the aorta to become the thoracic duct. It passes behind the carotid sheath at the level of C7 vertebra. It also passes behind the first part of the subclavian artery, and ascends first behind and then to the left of the oesophagus. The duct empties into the venous system of the neck at the union of the internal jugular and subclavian veins.

8. A

The median nerve arises from the lateral and medial cords of the brachial plexus (C6–8, T1). It gives off no branches in the arm. It supplies the radial half of the flexor digitorum profundus (the ulnar nerve supplies the ulnar half), the first (lateral) two lumbricals, the thenar eminence muscles and sensation to the lateral three and a half fingers (palmar aspect). (See figure accompanying answer to Question 5 above.)

9. B C D

The biceps brachialis, which is the chief supinator, is innervated by the musculocutaneous nerve (C5, C6). The ulnar nerve supplies the flexor carpi ulnaris and the medial half of the flexor digitorum profundus. The small hand muscles are responsible for the opposition of the thumb or splaying of the fingers, and are supplied by the ulnar nerve (T1). The peroneal branch of the sciatic nerve (C4, C5) supplies the anterior tibial muscle which is responsible for ankle dorsiflexion.

10. B D

The sole of the foot is innervated by S1, the groin by L1, and the index finger by C7.

11. E

The CSF is contained in the subarachnoid space. Pain and temperature sensation are transmitted through the anterior spinothalamic tracts, whereas proprioception, vibration and 2-point discrimination are transmitted through the posterior columns. The cord extends from the foramen magnum and ends in the filum terminale at the level of L2, L3. Hemisection causes an ipsilateral paralysis below the level of the lesion.

12. A C D

The main connections between the portal and systemic venous systems include:

1. Oesophageal branch of the left gastric veins and the oesophageal veins of the azygos system.
2. Inferior mesenteric vein of the portal system and the inferior haemorrhoidal veins draining into the internal iliac veins.
3. Portal tributaries in the mesentery and mesocolon and the retroperitoneal veins communicating with the renal, lumbar and phrenic veins.
4. Portal branches in the liver and the veins of the anterior abdominal

wall via veins passing along the falciform ligament to the umbilicus.
5. Portal branches in the liver and the veins of the diaphragm across the bare area of the liver.

13. D

The common peroneal (lateral popliteal) nerve supplies the anterior compartment muscles of the leg, which turn the foot upwards and outwards. It provides sensation to the anterolateral aspect of the lower half of the leg, including the ankle and dorsum of the foot. The common peroneal nerve is more susceptible to injury than the tibial nerve. It results in foot drop with paralysis of dorsiflexion or foot eversion and toe extension. There is sensory loss to the anterolateral aspect of the lower half of the leg, e.g. tibial nerve damage results in a claw-like deformity of the toes, and loss of sensation to the sole of the foot. In an equinovarus deformity, the foot is plantar-flexed and inverted. The opposite to that is called calcaneovalgus and is a feature of a tibial nerve injury.

14. B D

The facial nerve gives off the chorda tympani 5 mm above the stylomastoid foramen. The forehead muscles are spared in upper motor neurone lesions, since these muscles receive bilateral cortical fibres. If the intracranial part of the nerve is involved there is loss of taste over the anterior two-thirds of the tongue, due to involvement of the chorda tympani nerve, and hyperacusis due to paralysis of the stapedius muscle.

15. D

In S1 root lesions, there is paraesthesia over the lateral aspect of the foot, impairment of the ankle jerk and weakness of the plantar flexors of the foot.

16. A B C

At the lower end of the oesophagus the azygos tributaries (systemic) communicate with tributaries of the left gastric vein (portal). The thoracic part of the oesophagus lies posterior to the recurrent laryngeal nerve. It extends from the lower border of the cricoid cartilage (C6) to the level of the 10th thoracic vertebra. About 50% of carcinomas of the oesophagus occur in the middle third and 25% occur in the lower third. Distal oesophageal carcinomas are more likely to be due to adenocarcinoma.

17. C E

The radial nerve arises from the main branch of the posterior cord of the brachial plexus (C5–8). It supplies the extensor muscles of the forearm, wrist, finger and thumb. The biceps muscle is innervated by the musculocutaneous nerve. Radial nerve injury in the arm results in a wrist drop, atrophy of the triceps and paraesthesia of the dorsum of the hand between the 1st and 2nd metacarpals. Median nerve damage at the elbow results in loss of pronation at the elbow.

18. A C E

The internal jugular vein drains the cranial cavity and a few of the superficial veins of the head and neck. The internal jugular vein passes anterior to the thoracic duct on the left side and lies lateral to the internal and common carotid arteries within the carotid sheath.

19. B C D E

The follicular cells of the thyroid arise from epithelial proliferation at the base of the pharynx. The parafollicular cells which arise from the 5th pharyngeal pouch produce calcitonin.

20. D E

The IVC is formed behind the right common iliac artery by the right and left common iliac veins at the level of T12. It drains the veins of the abdomen, pelvis, lower extremities and azygous veins. It also receives the lumbar veins, the renal veins and the right inferior phrenic veins. The right suprarenal vein usually drains directly into the IVC, whereas the left one drains into the left renal vein.

21. C E

Damage to the T1 root, usually as a result of birth injury (e.g. traction with the arm extended), leads to a Klumpke's paralysis. An Erb–Duchenne paralysis results from damage to the C5, C6 roots. The main features of a Klumpke's paralysis are (i) paralysis of the intrinsic hand muscles ('claw hand'), (ii) sensory loss over the medial border of the forearm and hand, and over the medial two fingers, and (iii) Horner's syndrome due to traction on the sympathetic chain. Elbow flexion is mediated by the musculocutaneous nerve (C5 and C6) and pronation is mediated by C6 and C7 (lateral head of median nerve).

22. A B

The peroneus longus and the lateral tendons of the extensor digitorum longus assist in eversion. Flexor hallucis longus assists plantar flexion.

23. A E

Optic tract lesions result in a contralateral homonymous hemianopia. Lesions at the optic radiation in the temporal lobe result in a contralateral superior homonymous quadrantanopia. Contralateral inferior homonymous quadrantanopia results from lesions at the parietal part of the optic radiation.

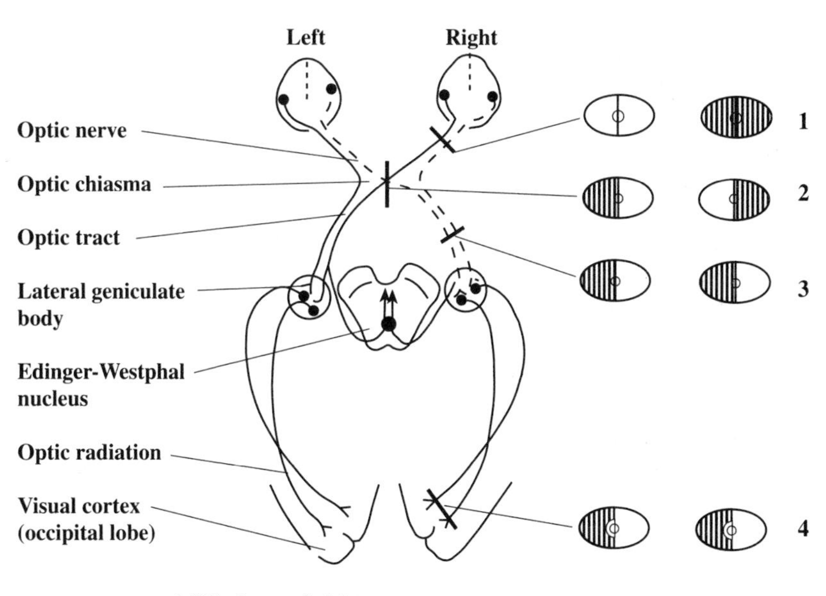

1. Blindness of right eye
2. Bitemporal hemianopia
3. Left homonymous hemianopia
4. Homonymous hemianopia with macular sparing (post-cerebral artery occlusion)

24. B C E

Broca's area is supplied by the middle cerebral artery. Wernicke's area is responsible for sensory speech. The anterior spinal arteries arise from the vertebral artery.

25. A B C

The following are features of an upper motor neurone lesion; weakness, spasticity, increased tendon reflexes, dissent abdominal reflexes and extensor plantar responses. With spinal cord lesion on the left side in the cervical region, there will be weakness of the arms and legs and an upgoing plantar on that side.

26. A B C

See figure accompanying answer to Question 23 above.

27. A C

Usually, a complete cord transection results from a spinal tumour (particularly extradural secondary deposits). As the neoplasm enlarges, it compresses the cord and induces ischaemia and infarction. In such cases, there is total loss of sensory modalities below the level of the lesion, since all sensory pathways are destroyed. There is also paralysis of all voluntary movements below the level of the lesion due to the destruction of the descending pathways. One to six weeks after transection reflex activity is regained and becomes exaggerated. The bladder and bowel function will be disturbed due to interruption of the descending autonomic fibres, and in particular to the parasympathetic nuclei in the S_3–S_5 segments.

6: PHYSIOLOGY

1. During the Valsalva manoeuvre, the following are observed:

- ☐ A a fall in jugular venous pressure (JVP)
- ☐ B tachycardia
- ☐ C increased stroke volume
- ☐ D a fall in systemic blood pressure
- ☐ E a rise in intrathoracic pressure

2. A high serum bicarbonate level of 38 mmol/l may be found in

- ☐ A pyloric stenosis
- ☐ B diabetic ketoacidosis
- ☐ C respiratory failure due to chronic bronchitis
- ☐ D ureterosigmoidostomy
- ☐ E renal tubular acidosis

3. Metabolic acidosis

- ☐ A may occur in bowel infarction
- ☐ B is associated with hyperkalaemia in renal tubular acidosis
- ☐ C cannot be present if the arterial pH is normal
- ☐ D is expressed by a fall in the standard bicarbonate level
- ☐ E the major compensatory change is an increased production of bicarbonate by renal tubular cells

4. Acute blood loss of 1.5 litres leads to a decrease in

- ☐ A the rate of oxygen extraction by peripheral tissues
- ☐ B the firing rate of carotid and aortic baroreceptors
- ☐ C renin secretion
- ☐ D the platelet count
- ☐ E the cardiac output

5. The consequences of resection of the terminal ileum include

- ☐ A subacute combined degeneration of the spinal cord
- ☐ B diarrhoea
- ☐ C decreased incidence of gallstone formation
- ☐ D iron deficiency anaemia (assuming no bleeding at anastomosis)
- ☐ E peripheral neuropathy

6. The consequences of biventricular failure include

- ☐ A increased sympathetic outflow to the failing heart
- ☐ B increased venous pressure
- ☐ C decreased activity of the renin–angiotensin–aldosterone system
- ☐ D shifting of normal Starling curve in an upward direction
- ☐ E accumulation of salt and water in the interstitial space

7. With respect to control of respiration

- ☐ A the inspiratory neurons are located in the midbrain
- ☐ B hypoxia increases the firing of the carotid bodies
- ☐ C increased arterial pCO_2 increases ventilation mainly by stimulating the central chemoreceptors
- ☐ D an increase in arterial H^+ concentration not due to increased pCO_2 increases ventilation mainly by stimulating the central chemoreceptors
- ☐ E in patients with chronic obstructive airways disease, hypoxia rather than hypercapnia is the main stimulus to ventilation

8. Airflow limitation leads to a reduction in

- ☐ A the forced expiratory volume in one second (FEV_1)
- ☐ B the ratio of FEV_1 to forced vital capacity (FVC)
- ☐ C residual volume
- ☐ D the ventilation perfusion ratio (i.e. $V/Q<1$)
- ☐ E the peak expiratory flow rate (PEFR)

9. The following statements about investigations used in respiratory disease are correct:

- ☐ A when performing a perfusion scan, macro-aggregated labelled human albumin remains in the pulmonary capillaries for a few hours
- ☐ B xenon-133 gas can be used to perform a ventilation scan
- ☐ C the gas transfer factor reflects the uptake of O_2 from the alveolus into the red cell
- ☐ D the gas transfer factor is independent of the thickness of the alveolar membrane
- ☐ E the gas transfer factor is usually increased in severe emphysema

10. Cortisol

- ☐ A synthesis by the adrenals is controlled by ACTH via cyclic AMP
- ☐ B reduces gluconeogenesis
- ☐ C plasma level reaches a maximum at about midnight
- ☐ D has some mineralocorticoid activity
- ☐ E enhances production of angiotensinogen

11. The initial consequences of acute upper airway obstruction include

- ☐ A cyanosis
- ☐ B bradycardia
- ☐ C a rise in blood pH
- ☐ D polycythaemia
- ☐ E inspiratory stridor

12. Consider the following diagram representing subdivisions of the lung volume

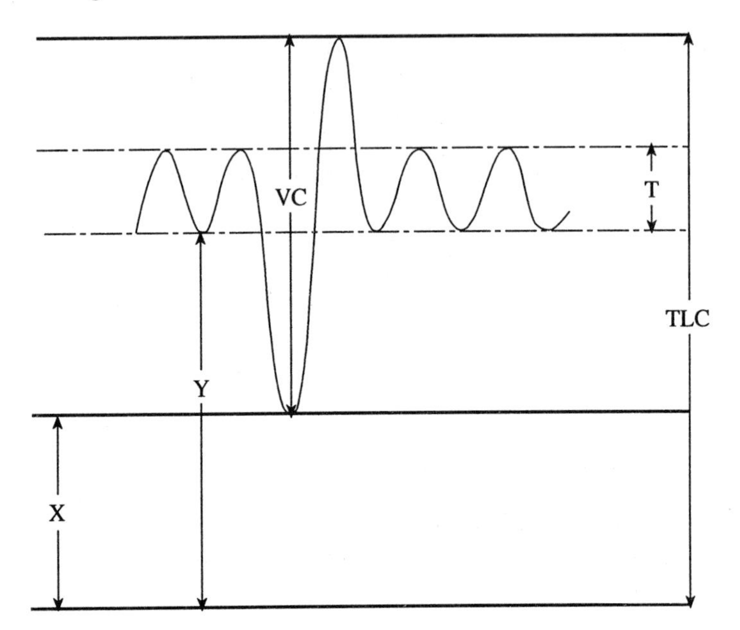

T = resting tidal volume; VC = vital capacity; TLC = total lung capacity; X and Y represent volumes.

- ☐ A X is the functional residual capacity
- ☐ B Y is the expiratory reserve volume
- ☐ C TLC can be measured using a simple spirometer
- ☐ D a general anaesthetic increases Y
- ☐ E X is increased in a patient with emphysema

13. Considering the ABO and rhesus (Rh) systems

- ☐ A if the patient's blood group is AB, his serum will have the naturally occurring anti-A and anti-B antibodies
- ☐ B naturally occurring anti-A and anti-B antibodies are usually IgG
- ☐ C less than 10% of Caucasians are rhesus positive
- ☐ D the presence of the D antigen makes the subject rhesus positive
- ☐ E rhesus antibodies are naturally occurring antibodies

14. The following are characteristics of erythropoiesis and erythropoietin:

- ☐ A hypoxia is the main stimulus to erythropoietin production
- ☐ B bilateral nephrectomy completely abolishes erythropoietin activity
- ☐ C erythropoietin increases the maturation time of red blood cell precursors
- ☐ D erythropoietin stimulates δ-aminolaevulinate synthetase (ALA-S) activity in red blood cell precursors
- ☐ E erythropoietin levels are found to be low in polycythaemia rubra vera

15. The following statements about the control of the peripheral circulation and blood pressure are correct:

- ☐ A the arterioles account for about 40% of total peripheral resistance
- ☐ B carotid chemoreceptors have no role in blood pressure control
- ☐ C the central vasomotor centre is situated in the medulla oblongata
- ☐ D the sudden assumption of an upright posture increases the discharge rate from the carotid and aortic baroreceptors
- ☐ E the sudden assumption of an upright posture causes constriction of the medium-sized veins

16. Vasoactive intestinal polypeptide (VIP)

☐ A is secreted by non-beta islet cells in the pancreas
☐ B stimulates gastric acid secretion
☐ C enhances small intestinal reabsorption of water and electrolytes
☐ D normal serum level is 3000 pg/ml
☐ E may be secreted by a bronchogenic carcinoma

17. The following statements about vitamin K are true:

☐ A fat malabsorption is the commonest cause of vitamin K deficiency in adults
☐ B none of the available preparations can be absorbed in the absence of bile salts
☐ C it functions as a biological antioxidant
☐ D vitamin K reverses warfarin effects almost instantaneously
☐ E warfarin inhibits the vitamin K-dependent carboxylation of factors I, V and XI in the liver

18. Following trauma to a blood vessel

☐ A the platelets immediately adhere to subendothelial fibres
☐ B platelet aggregation is induced by ADP and thrombin
☐ C minute ruptures in small vessels are often sealed by a platelet plug rather than by a blood clot
☐ D the vessel wall endothelium produces thromboxane A2 which inhibits platelet adhesion
☐ E low dose aspirin does not affect the synthesis of thromboxane A2

19. The following occur in the successfully sympathectomized left hand:

☐ A the permanent abolition of sweating
☐ B the skin does not respond to central temperature changes
☐ C the skin does not respond to local temperature changes
☐ D the large increase in blood flow following the operation is well maintained for years
☐ E if the skin is ischaemic, the ischaemia may improve

20. The following factors stimulate ADH (vasopressin) secretion:

- ☐ A exercise
- ☐ B alcohol
- ☐ C severe hypovolaemia
- ☐ D decreased plasma osmolarity
- ☐ E pain

21. The following statements about bilirubin and its metabolites are correct:

- ☐ A the daily production of bilirubin in a 70 kg adult is about 300 mg
- ☐ B the conjugation of bilirubin is catalyzed by the enzyme β-glucuronidase
- ☐ C conjugated bilirubin is secreted into the bile by simple diffusion
- ☐ D a fraction of urobilinogen is reabsorbed from the intestine and re-excreted through the liver
- ☐ E urobilins are colourless compounds

22. The following statements about potassium homoeostasis in the body are correct:

- ☐ A 20% of the total body potassium is located in the extracellular compartment
- ☐ B aldosterone increases active potassium secretion in the distal convoluted tubule
- ☐ C hypokalaemia directly stimulates aldosterone secretion
- ☐ D hypokalaemia will result if the activity of the membrane-bound, ATP-dependent sodium pump is impaired
- ☐ E insulin causes potassium to enter the cell

23. The following statements about CO_2 in the blood are correct:

☐ A for a given pH, the partial pressure of CO_2 (pCO_2) is inversely proportional to the bicarbonate concentration [HCO_3^-]
☐ B most of the CO_2 in the blood is present in the form of carbonic acid H_2CO_3
☐ C CO_2 diffuses into red blood cells in the capillary beds
☐ D haemoglobin is the main buffer for H^+ generated by the entry of CO_2 into red blood cells
☐ E pCO_2 is usually higher than normal in compensated metabolic alkalosis

24. The following statements about hydrogen ion homoeostasis (H^+) are correct:

☐ A bicarbonate is the most important buffer in the extracellular fluid
☐ B proteins are the principal buffer in urine
☐ C hydrogen ions are secreted into the renal tubular lumen in exchange for potassium ions (K^+), and combine with the filtered bicarbonate
☐ D ammonium ions (NH_4^+) cross the membranes of renal tubular cells
☐ E the hydrogen ion concentration is directly proportional to the partial pressure of CO_2

25. The following statements about the measurement of the GFR are correct:

☐ A creatinine clearance is higher than the true GFR
☐ B creatinine clearance is directly proportional to serum creatinine concentration
☐ C the GFR can be calculated from the rate of fall in the level of radioactivity after the injection of ^{51}Cr-labelled EDTA
☐ D serum urea is a more accurate index of GFR than serum creatinine
☐ E inulin clearance is used to estimate GFR in routine clinical practice

26. With respect to the nephron in a healthy kidney

- ☐ A the descending loop of Henlé is impermeable to water
- ☐ B almost all the filtered protein is reabsorbed in the proximal convoluted tubule
- ☐ C ADH renders the cells lining the collecting ducts permeable to water
- ☐ D in the distal tubule, further Na^+ is reabsorbed, whereas K^+ and H^+ are secreted under the influence of ADH (vasopressin)
- ☐ E all the filtered glucose is reabsorbed in the proximal tubule

27. A good assessment of GFR is provided by the following:

- ☐ A serum albumin
- ☐ B serum creatinine
- ☐ C serum B_2-microglobulin (in a healthy subject)
- ☐ D water deprivation test
- ☐ E amino acid chromatography on urine

28. The following are increased in the presence of hypoglycaemia:

- ☐ A glucagon secretion
- ☐ B epinephrine output from the adrenal medulla
- ☐ C glucokinase activity
- ☐ D growth hormone secretion by the anterior pituitary
- ☐ E cortisol secretion

29. The oxygen dissociation curve is shifted to the right with

- ☐ A pyrexia
- ☐ B respiratory acidosis
- ☐ C states of decreased concentration of 2,3-DPG inside the red cell
- ☐ D polycythaemia
- ☐ E sickle cell anaemia

30. The following statements about hormones and pregnancy are correct:

- ☐ A human chorionic gonadotrophin (hCG) becomes undetectable in urine in the third trimester
- ☐ B the synthesis of human placental lactogen (hPL) is dependent on both placental and fetal enzymes
- ☐ C pregnanediol is the main urinary metabolite of progesterone
- ☐ D a low serum progesterone in pregnancy is associated with recurrent abortions
- ☐ E the fetal liver and adrenals take part in the synthesis of oestriol

31. The principal actions of insulin include

- ☐ A increased lipolysis in adipose tissue
- ☐ B increased ketogenesis in the liver
- ☐ C increased glucose uptake by muscle and adipose tissue
- ☐ D decreased glycogen synthesis
- ☐ E increased protein synthesis

32. When the renin–angiotensin system is stimulated by hypovolaemic shock

- ☐ A renin converts angiotensin I into angiotensin II
- ☐ B angiotensin II causes vasoconstriction of the efferent glomerular arteriole
- ☐ C angiotensin I stimulates the adrenal medulla to synthesize aldosterone
- ☐ D angiotensin II stimulates the adrenal cortex to increase cortisol production
- ☐ E angiotensin converting enzymes degrade bradykinin

33. The following factors stimulate renin release:

☐ A a decrease in blood pressure
☐ B propranolol
☐ C an increase in plasma K^+ concentration
☐ D angiotensin II
☐ E salt depletion

34. The blood–brain barrier

☐ A contains endothelial cells which have tight junctions
☐ B allows transport of substances in one direction only, i.e. from the vascular system into the brain
☐ C allows water to cross by simple diffusion
☐ D contains astrocytic foot processes
☐ E lacks mitochondria in the endothelial cells

35. The normal CSF contains

☐ A about 10 polymorphs per mm^3
☐ B oligoclonal bands in approximately 50% of the general population
☐ C 0.2–0.4 g per litre of protein
☐ D immunoglobulin (IgG)
☐ E less than one-third of blood glucose

36. The electromyogram (EMG)

☐ A records the electrical activity of muscle fibres making up the motor units
☐ B records the magnitude of muscle contraction
☐ C shows regular electrical activity when healthy muscle is relaxed
☐ D can be recorded by placing the electrode on the skin overlying the muscle
☐ E shows fibrillation potentials in denervated muscle

37. The diagram below represents an action potential recorded from an unmyelinated axon

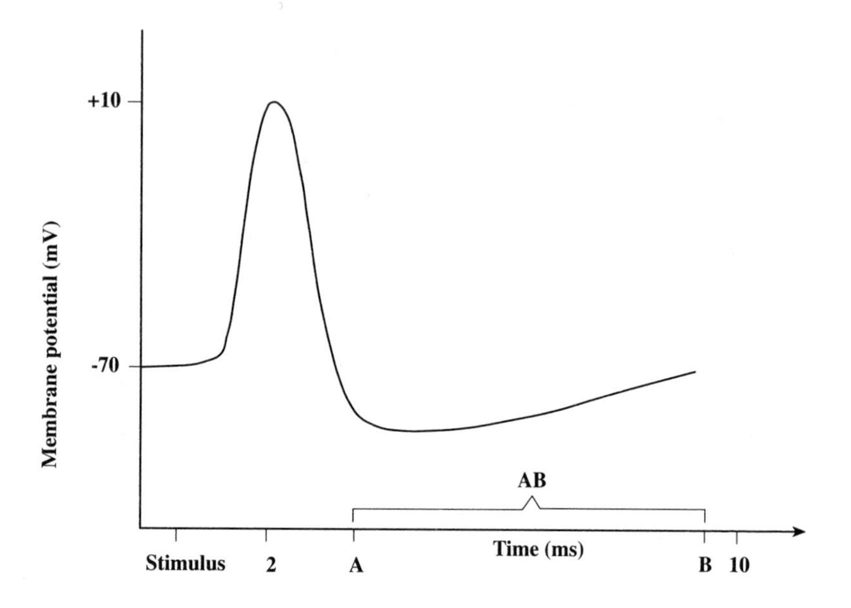

☐ A during AB phase hyperpolarization the Na^+ channels are more active than the K^+ channels
☐ B during AB a stronger current (stimulus) is needed to generate another action potential
☐ C more ionic exchange (across the membrane) occurs in this unmyelinated axon than in a myelinated axon
☐ D the greater the diameter of the axon, the greater the conduction velocity of this action potential
☐ E saltatory conduction is a feature of conduction in unmyelinated axons

38. The following factors decrease cerebral blood flow (CBF):

- ☐ A seizures
- ☐ B inhalation of 7% CO_2
- ☐ C intraventricular administration of norepinephrine
- ☐ D chronic anaemia
- ☐ E inhalation of hyperbaric oxygen

39. The spinothalamic tracts of the spinal cord transmit the following sensory modalities:

- ☐ A pain
- ☐ B two point discrimination
- ☐ C joint position
- ☐ D temperature
- ☐ E vibration

40. The following autonomic neurons are adrenergic:

- ☐ A postganglion sympathetic neurons to the small bowel
- ☐ B postganglion sympathetic neurons to the sweat glands
- ☐ C autonomic preganglionic neurons
- ☐ D the parasympathetic fibres supplying the sphincter pupillae of the iris
- ☐ E postganglionic parasympathetic neurons to the stomach

41. Cholinergic impulses in the autonomic nervous system produce

- ☐ A a decrease in atrial contractility
- ☐ B detrusor muscle relaxation
- ☐ C ciliary muscle contraction
- ☐ D gallbladder relaxation
- ☐ E ejaculation

42. The following factors stimulate gastrin secretion:

☐ A increased vagal activity
☐ B hypercalcaemia
☐ C increased gastric acidity
☐ D secretin
☐ E a protein meal

43. The following statements about the electrocardiogram are correct:

☐ A opening of the aortic valve coincides with the P wave
☐ B isovolumetric contraction occurs during the P wave
☐ C during the ST segment, all parts of ventricles have been depolarized
☐ D the QT interval may be prolonged in hypokalaemia
☐ E during the T wave, the tricuspid valve is normally closed

44. The following are acceptable methods for reducing intracranial pressure:

☐ A hypoventilation
☐ B intravenous mannitol
☐ C the administration of atracurium
☐ D the administration of sodium nitroprusside
☐ E positioning the patient in the head down position

45. The following transmitter substances increase intestinal secretion of water and electrolytes:

☐ A noradrenaline
☐ B VIP (vasoactive intestinal polypeptide)
☐ C prostaglandins
☐ D dihydroxy bile acids
☐ E acetylcholine

46. In the digestion and absorption of fat

☐ A a low pH enhances pancreatic lipase action
☐ B vitamins A, D, E and K are packaged into the chylomicrons within the enterocytes
☐ C bile salts act as emulsifying agents
☐ D deficiency of apoprotein B synthesis causes fat malabsorption
☐ E long-chain triglycerides are more water-soluble than medium-chain triglycerides (MCTs)

47. Nociception (pain)

☐ A is transmitted faster through C fibres than through A fibres
☐ B is transmitted through the dorsal columns of the spinal cord
☐ C of visceral origin is poorly localized and nauseating in character
☐ D transmission is facilitated by the stimulation of μ receptors in the CNS
☐ E in disseminated cancer, may be relieved by lobotomy

48. The luteinizing hormone releasing hormone (LHRH)

☐ A has a constant secretion rate throughout the day
☐ B controls the secretion of FSH
☐ C analogues may be used in the treatment of prostatic carcinoma
☐ D may be used in the treatment of infertility in both sexes
☐ E produces a greater response in LH release when given intravenously during the early follicular phase than during the luteal phase

49. The following statements about the mechanism of vomiting are correct:

☐ A the main receptors in the chemoreceptor trigger zone (CTZ) are dopaminergic (D2)
☐ B the CTZ is not protected by the blood–brain barrier
☐ C $5HT_3$ (hydroxytryptamine) agonists are effective anti-emetics in cis-platinum-induced vomiting
☐ D anticholinergic drugs inhibit vomiting by acting mainly on CTZ
☐ E stimulation of H_1 receptors in the vestibular system inhibits vomiting

50. Adult haemoglobin

☐ A contains four molecules of globin
☐ B combines with carbon dioxide
☐ C combines with carbon monoxide at the same site on the haemoglobin molecule as oxygen
☐ D carries molecular rather than ionic oxygen
☐ E production is increased by the direct action of hypoxia on the bone marrow

51. The QRS complex on the electrocardiogram

☐ A is caused by ventricular myocardial repolarization
☐ B will normally contain a Q-wave up to half the height of the R wave
☐ C corresponds to the phase of isovolumetric contraction
☐ D is shortened in tricyclic poisoning
☐ E may be used to assess the rotation of the heart along its longitudinal axis

52. In respiratory muscle weakness involving the intercostal muscles and diaphragm

- ☐ A the ratio of forced expiratory volume in one second (FEV_1) to vital capacity (VC) is reduced
- ☐ B the ratio of residual volume (RV) to total lung capacity (TLC) is increased
- ☐ C gas transfer (corrected for lung volume) is reduced
- ☐ D hypercapnia is an early feature
- ☐ E the VC falls when the patient is moved from an upright to a supine position

53. The following cause vasodilatation of the peripheral arterial blood vessels:

- ☐ A endothelin
- ☐ B nitric oxide
- ☐ C prostaglandins
- ☐ D thromboxane A2
- ☐ E adenosine diphosphate

ANSWERS AND TEACHING NOTES: PHYSIOLOGY

1. **B D E**

The Valsalva manoeuvre refers to forced expiration against a closed glottis. The resulting increase in intrapulmonary and intrathoracic pressures impedes venous return. This causes a decreased stroke volume and blood pressure. On release, there is a transient increase in peripheral volume leading to an overshoot of blood pressure and a decreased heart rate.

2. **A C**

Actual bicarbonate level = 23–33 mmol/l. An elevated plasma [HCO_3^-] can result from metabolic alkalosis or the secondary metabolic response to respiratory acidosis. The projectile vomiting of pyloric stenosis results in H^+ loss and metabolic alkalosis. Other causes of a metabolic alkalosis include excess oral intake of alkali or forced alkaline diuresis and thiazide or loop diuretic therapy. Metabolic acidosis (low serum HCO_3) is a feature of diabetic ketoacidosis, ureterosigmoidostomy and renal tubular acidosis.

3. **A B D**

The addition of acids stronger than buffer acids to the blood, results in a metabolic acidosis. This stimulates the respiratory system in order to excrete CO_2:

$$H^+ + HCO_3 <> H_2CO_3 \longrightarrow H_2O + CO_2$$

This respiratory compensation reduces serum HCO_3 and elevates pH which could rise to normal levels. The renal compensatory mechanisms then bring about the excretion of extra H^+ and return the buffer systems to normal.

4. **B E**

Hypovolaemia results in hypotension. The decrease in systemic blood pressure results in inhibition of baroreceptors (in order to increase peripheral resistance) and an increase in renin secretion. The latter increases the availability of angiotensins (vasopressors) and aldosterone (Na^+ and water retention). The cardiac output falls and the platelet count rises.

5. **A B E**

The terminal ileum is the site for absorption of vitamin B12 and bile salts. Vitamin B12 deficiency may result in subacute degeneration of the spinal cord and a peripheral neuropathy. The decrease in bile salt reabsorption increases the incidence of gallstones and reduces fat digestion and absorption. Diarrhoea results from fatty stools, colonic irritation by bile salts and a shorter small bowel.

6. A B E

The reduced cardiac output stimulates the sympathetic system via the baroreceptors. The decreased renal perfusion stimulates the renin–angiotensin–aldosterone system which increases vasoconstriction and water and salt retention. There is widespread vasoconstriction. The Starling curve moves downwards when the heart fails.

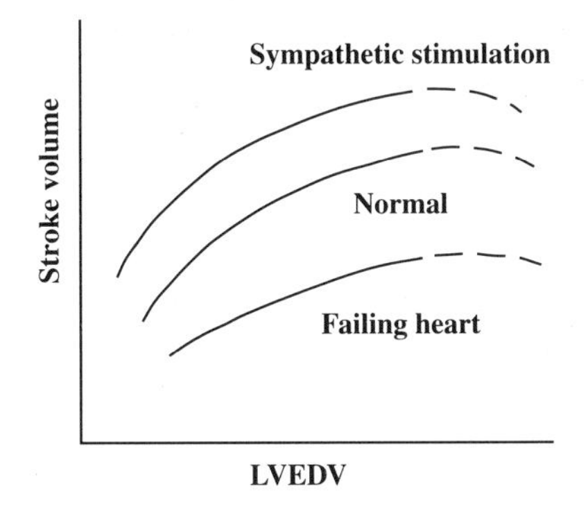

7. B C E

The central regulatory centres that control the rate and depth of respiration are located in the medulla and pons. The carotid body chemoreceptors respond to decreases in arterial pO_2, high pCO_2 and low pH. The aortic body chemoreceptors respond to increased levels of pCO_2 and low pO_2. CO_2 stimulates the central chemoreceptors by an increase of pCO_2 (H^+) in the CSF. Hypoxia is the main stimulus to respiratory drive in patients with chronic obstructive airway disease.

8. A B D E

Airflow limitation reduces FEV_1, FEV_1/FVC, V/Q and PEFR. Patients with obstructive lung disease have a large total lung capacity, and a reduced vital capacity because their residual volume is increased.

9. A B C

The ventilation pattern of the lungs can be assessed by having the patient inhale ^{133}Xe while monitoring the chest with radiation detectors. The gas transfer factor depends on the thickness of the alveolar membrane. It is decreased in diffuse infiltrative lung disorders, pulmonary fibrosis, multiple pulmonary emboli and emphysema. It is increased in asthma, hyperkinetic states, left to right shunts and polycythaemia.

10. A D E

ACTH binds to special receptors on the plasma membrane of adrenocortical cells causing an increase in intracellular cAMP and activation of protein kinase A. Cortisol has a circadian rhythm and is highest in the morning (around 8.00 am) and lowest around midnight. Cortisol has several anti-insulin actions, including stimulation of glycogenesis (liver) and gluconeogenesis from protein (liver). It also increases protein catabolism, lipolysis and free fatty acid mobilization, and has some mineralocorticoid action.

11. A E

Asphyxia results in hypercapnia and hypoxia simultaneously. This stimulates the respiratory system vigorously. Initially there is tachycardia and hypertension with high levels of catecholamines, but later bradycardia and hypotension supervene.

12. E

X is the residual volume, Y is the functional residual capacity. TLC is measured using helium dilution. The residual volume is usually increased in emphysema.

13. D

The naturally occurring antibodies are usually IgM. Rhesus antibodies are immune antibodies. Approximately 80% of Caucasians are rhesus positive, whereas Africans and Japanese are generally rhesus negative. A subject whose blood group is AB does not have anti-A and anti-B antibodies in the serum.

14. A D E

Hypoxia is the chief stimulus to erythropoiesis. 85% of erythropoietin (166 amino acids) is produced by the kidneys and 15% is produced by the liver. The rate controlling enzyme for porphyrin and haem synthesis is ALA-S. Its synthesis is inhibited by Hb in polycythaemia rubra vera. Genetically engineered erythropoietin is now available for the treatment of anaemia caused by renal failure.

15. A C E

Hypoxia stimulates the carotid chemoreceptors causing tachycardia and vasoconstriction and an elevation in blood pressure. Sudden assumption of the upright posture results in a fall in venous return, stroke volume, cardiac output and blood pressure. This stimulates the sympathetic system which causes constriction of medium-sized veins and a decrease in the firing rate of the carotid and aortic baroreceptors (stretch receptors). The compensatory response is an increase in heart rate and peripheral resistance.

16. A E

VIP (28 amino acids) stimulates the intestinal secretion of water and electrolytes. It inhibits gastric acid secretion and causes peripheral vasodilatation. VIPomas result in the Werner–Morrison or WDHA syndrome (watery diarrhoea, hypokalaemia and achlorhydria).

17. A B

Vitamin K is a fat-soluble vitamin and deficiency occurs in fat-malabsorption states. Warfarin inhibits vitamin K epoxide reductase, thereby inhibiting the formation of the reduced form of vitamin K (KH_2). This reduced form is the cofactor for decarboxylation of glutamate residues in the inactive proenzyme forms of factors X, IX, VII and II in the liver. It takes approximately 21 hours for vitamin K to reverse warfarin effects.

18. A B C

Injury to the wall of a blood vessel causes contraction and platelet aggregation. This temporary haemostatic plug is converted to a definitive plug by thrombin. The vascular endothelium produces prostacyclin which inhibits platelet adhesion.

19. A B E

Interruption of the sympathetic nerve supply abolishes sweating and the skin response to central temperature changes. The vasodilation following sympathectomy causes an initial increase of blood flow, but this increase is not usually maintained permanently.

20. A C E

Stimuli to ADH secretion include: increased osmotic pressure of the plasma, emotional stress, surgical trauma, pain, morphine, nicotine and barbiturates. Release of ADH can occur in response to an increase in osmolarity (via stimulation of osmoreceptors located in the anterior hypothalamus) or a decreased fluid volume (via a decrease in the stretch of the volume receptors located in the left atrium, vena cavae, carotid sinus and aortic arch).

21. A D

Bilirubin is formed from the catabolism of the haem moeity of haemoglobin, and is transported to the liver bound to albumin. Bilirubin is conjugated with glucuronic acid catalysed by glucuronyl transferase to form water-soluble bilirubin diglucuronide which is excreted into the bile canaliculi via an active process. The conjugated bilirubin is converted by intestinal bacteria into unconjugated bilirubin and urobilinogens (colourless compounds) which are reabsorbed by intestinal mucosa. Some of the reabsorbed substances are re-excreted by the liver (enterohepatic circulation).

22. B E

Only about 2% of body potassium is located in the extracellular compartment. Hyperkalaemia stimulates aldosterone secretion which increases potassium secretion in the distal tubule. Impairment of the sodium pump causes K^+ to accumulate extracellularly, whereas insulin causes K^+ to enter cells.

23. C D E

Most of the carbon dioxide in the blood is present in the form of bicarbonate (HCO_3). The partial pressure of CO_2 is directly proportional to the concentration of HCO_3:

$$pCO_2 = pH \times K \times [HCO_3^-]$$

The respiratory system can compensate for metabolic alkalosis by retaining CO_2 in order to restore blood pH.

24. A E

Phosphate is the main buffer in urine, whereas HCO_3^- is the main buffer in the blood. H^+ are secreted into the renal tubular lumen in exchange for

Na^+. NH_4^+ cannot cross cell membranes because of the electrical charge, whereas NH_3 can. The H^+ concentration is related to $[HCO_3^-]$ and pCO_2 through the following relationship:

$$[H^+] = K \frac{pCO_2}{[HCO_3^-]}$$

25. A C

Creatinine clearance is inversely proportional to the serum creatinine concentration and is higher than true GFR due to active secretion of creatinine in the renal tubules. Creatinine clearance is used conventionally in clinical practice to estimate GFR. Serum urea concentration is influenced by many factors and therefore it is a less accurate index than serum creatinine.

26. B C E

The ascending loop of Henlé is impermeable to water. Aldosterone (and not ADH) controls Na^+ reabsorption in exchange for H^+ and K^+ in the distal tubule.

27. B C

The water deprivation test assesses distal tubular function, whereas amino acid chromatography assesses proximal tubular function.

28. A B D E

Glucagon acts on hepatocytes and increases intracellular cAMP and cytoplasmic Ca^{2+}, thereby stimulating glycogenolysis. Hypoglycaemia also stimulates the release of catecholamines, TSH, glucocorticoids and growth hormone.

29. A B E

The oxygen dissociation curve is shifted to the right by a high pCO_2, raised temperature, acidosis, and 2,3-diphosphoglycerate (2,3-DPG), such that a higher pO_2 is required to bind a given amount of oxygen. Production of 2,3-DPG is stimulated by hypoxia due to anaemia and altitude. The oxygen dissociation curve is pushed to the left by a low concentration of 2,3-DPG, a low pCO_2, acute alkalosis, hypothermia and certain rare haemoglobinopathies, with oxyhaemoglobin and carboxyhaemoglobin.

30. C D E

Although hCG hormone begins to fall around the 11th week of pregnancy, it remains detectable. Fetal enzymes are involved in the synthesis of oestriol but not hPL.

31. C E

Insulin decreases lipolysis and ketogenesis and increases glycogen synthesis and glucose uptake by cells. It also has an anabolic effect on proteins. (See also the answers and teaching notes to Question 8, Chapter 7, Clinical Chemistry.)

32. B E

Renin converts angiotensin into angiotensin I. The latter is converted into angiotensin II by the converting enzyme. Angiotensin II is vasoactive and stimulates aldosterone secretion and depresses renin output.

The renin-angiotensin system

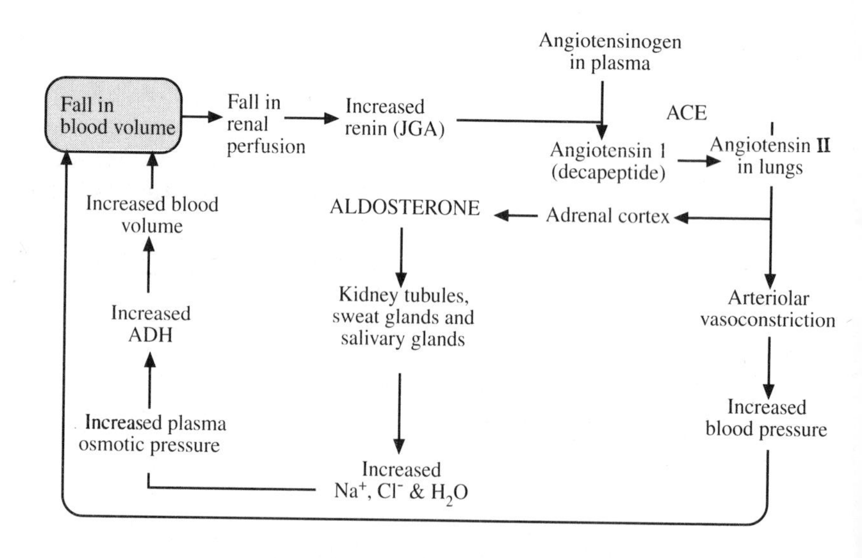

33. A E

A decrease in the circulating blood volume, potassium depletion, catecholamines and oral contraceptives stimulate renin secretion, whereas angiotensin II, ADH, hypernatraemia and hyperkalaemia, ACE inhibitors and β-blockers reduce renin release. Renin effectively raises blood pressure and blood volume.

34. A C D

The blood–brain barrier allows lipid soluble substances, oxygen, CO_2 and water to cross easily, whereas water-soluble ones cross with difficulty. The transport process may be in both directions. Its endothelial cells have six times the number of mitochondria as other endothelial cells.

35. C D

The normal CSF contains mononuclear cells only (5 per mm^3). The presence of oligoclonal bands may indicate CNS disease, e.g. multiple sclerosis. It contains 0.2–0.4 g/l of protein and the glucose concentration should be greater than 50% of that in the blood. The presence of low glucose concentration is found in bacterial, fungal and tuberculous meningitis.

36. B C D

During the hyperpolarization phase, the K^+ channels are more active than the Na^+ channels. Ionic exchange in myelinated axons occurs mainly at the nodes of Ranvier. This means that less metabolic energy is required in myelinated fibres to pump the ions out once the impulse has passed. Increased axon diameter and myelination increase conduction velocity. Saltatory conduction is seen in myelinated fibres where the electrical impulse leaps (=saltare) from one node to another.

37. A D E

The EMG which records the electrical activity of muscle fibres does not reflect the magnitude of muscle contraction and shows no regular electrical activity in relaxed healthy muscle.

38. E

Seizures, hypercapnia, intraventricular norepinephrine and chronic anaemia increase CBF. Other factors which increase CBF include local acidosis and hypoxia. A local increase in pO_2 or a decrease in pCO_2 have a vasoconstrictor effect on cerebral vessels.

39. A D

Two point discrimination, proprioception and vibration sensation travel through the posterior columns, whereas pain and temperature are transmitted through the spinothalamic tracts.

40. A

Postganglion sympathetic neurons to the sweat glands, autonomic preganglionic neurons, and parasympathetic fibres to smooth muscle are cholinergic.

41. A C

Parasympathetic stimulation decreases atrial contractility and causes the contraction of the detrusor muscle, gall bladder and ciliary muscle (for near vision). Ejaculation is sympathetically mediated, whereas erection is a parasympathetic function.

System	**Parasympathetic**		**Sympathetic**	
	α_1	α_2	β_1	β_2
Heart	↓ rate ↓ atrial contractility ↓ AVN conduction		↑ rate and contractility ↑ AVN conduction ↑ renin secretion	
Vessels	Little effect	Vasoconstriction of arterioles (esp. skin, abdominal viscera and coronary circulation) Constriction of systemic veins		Vasodilation of coronary arterioles and in skeletal muscles
Bronchus	Bronchoconstriction			Bronchial muscle relaxation
Gut	↑ motility; relaxation of sphincters	↓ motility		↓ motility

System	**Parasympathetic**		**Sympathetic**	
	α_1	α_2	β_1	β_2
Pancreas	$\uparrow$ exocrine secretion No effect on β-cells of islets	$\downarrow$ exocrine secretion		$\uparrow$ endocrine secretion by β-cells; lipolysis; glycogenolysis gluconeo-genesis
Urogenital	Contraction of detrusor muscles of bladder; relaxation of sphincters	Relaxation of detrusor muscles; contraction of sphincters and pregnant uterus		Relaxation of pregnant uterus
Glands		$\uparrow$ secretion (lacrimal, salivary, alimentary)		$\uparrow$ secretion by sweat glands
Eye	Miosis-sphincter pupillae contracts			Mydriasis-dilator pupillae contracts

42. A B E

Gastrin is secreted by the antral G-cells. It increases gastric acid and pepsin secretion, stimulates insulin and glucagon secretion and gastric emptying. Stimuli for release include amino acids in the antrum, distension of the antrum by food and vagal action. Gastrin secretion is inhibited by a pH <1.5, gastric acid and secretin.

43. C D E

The opening of the aortic valve occurs during ventricular systole (QRS-T). Isovolumetric contraction also occurs during ventricular systole when the mitral and tricuspid valves are closed (it lasts for 0.05 seconds). Hypokalaemia causes prolongation of QT segment, ST depression and T wave inversion.

44. B C D

Hyperventilation reduces intracranial pressure (low pCO_2 causes cerebral vasoconstriction). Mannitol is an osmotic diuretic which reduces CSF volume. Atracurium is an anticholinergic drug which is a muscle relaxant and reduces intrathoracic and venous pressures. The head down position allows venous pooling into the cranium and raises intracranial pressure.

45. B C D E

Noradrenaline decreases intestinal secretion. Prostaglandins are thought to contribute to the diarrhoea caused by inflammatory bowel disease and radiation enteritis.

46. B C D

Pancreatic lipase is the most important enzyme in fat digestion. Deficiency of this enzyme due to pancreatic disease. Surgical resection leads to steatorrhea. Pancreatic lipase is more active in the presence of bicarbonate, therefore a low duodenal pH (as seen in gastrinoma) can also lead to steatorrhea. Lipids and bile salts interact to form micelles. Monoglycerides, cholesterol, and fatty acids from the micelles enter the mucosal cells by passive diffusion. The subsequent fate of the fatty acids depends on their size. Fatty acids containing less than 10–12 carbon atoms pass from the enterocytes directly into the portal blood. Fatty acids containing more than 10–12 carbon atoms are re-esterified to triglycerides within the mucosal cells. Chylomicrons containing triglycerides and cholesteryl esters enter the lymphatics and pass into the bloodstream through the thoracic duct.

47. C E

Transmission of pain is faster through myelinated fibres (A fibres). The dorsal columns relay position sense, vibration and touch. The spinothalamic tracts relay pain, temperature and touch. Visceral pain which is poorly localised may cause reflex contraction of nearby muscles. μ receptors are opiate receptors which mediate supraspinal analgesia, euphoria, dependence, gut stasis, meiosis and respirator depression. Other surgical procedures used to relieve intractable pain include sympathectomy, myelotomy, posterior rhizotomy, anterolateral cordotomy and thalatomy.

48. B C D

LHRH is secreted by the hypothalamus. It stimulates the release of FSH and LH by the anterior pituitary. The release of LHRH is pulsatile. Its analogues have been used recently in the treatment of prostatic and breast cancers, through down regulation of pituitary receptors, which decreases LH secretion.

49. A B

The chemoreceptor trigger zone is located on the lateral walls of the fourth ventricle and is more permeable to most substances than the underlying medulla. $5HT_3$ antagonists (e.g. Ondansetron) are effective against chemotherapy-induced vomiting. Anticholinergic drugs block muscarinic receptors in the vomiting centre and vestibular apparatus. Metoclopramide and phenothiazines act mainly on CTZ. Antihistamines are useful antiemetics.

50. B C D

Haemoglobin contains one molecule of globin which is bound to four haem molecules. The globin molecule comprises four polypeptide chains. Haemoglobin undergoes a reversible reaction with carbon monoxide to form carbaminohaemoglobin. Approximately 30% of carbon dioxide in the blood is carried in this form. The affinity of the haemoglobin binding site for carbon monoxide is 200-fold that of oxygen so that CO will displace O_2 from oxyhaemoglobin. Hypoxia is the main stimulus to increased production of haemoglobin, mediated by erythropoietin.

51. C E

The QRS complex is caused by ventricular depolarization. Ventricular repolarization is associated with the QT interval. The QRS complex corresponds to the process of isovolumetric contraction, when pressure in the ventricular cavities rises due to the onset of ventricular contraction. The pressure gradient across the atrioventricular (AV) valves is reversed, causing closure of the atrioventricular valve. After closure, the ventricular pressure rises to exceed that in the arteries, when ventricular ejection begins.

52. B E

Total lung capacity is reduced, and residual volume is increased because of reduction in inspiratory and expiratory capacity. Both of these factors reduce vital capacity, but because the FEV_1:VC ratio is normal there is no decrease in FEV_1. Hypercapnia is a late feature and usually does not appear until the VC has fallen to 50% of normal. The fall in the VC when the patient is moved from an upright to a supine position is a useful indicator of bilateral diaphragm weakness and paralysis. The patient becomes breathless on lying flat.

53. B C

Endothelin is a vasoconstricting peptide synthesized by endothelial cells and by neurones in the paraventricular nucleus of the hypothalamus. Nitric oxide is a potent vasodilator synthesized from L-arginine in vessel walls by NO synthases. In addition, inspired NO may be clinically useful as a vasodilator of pulmonary arteries. Iloprost (a prostacyclin PGI_2 analogue) may be beneficial in the treatment of the critically ischaemic limb. Both thromboxane A_2 and adenosine diphosphate cause vasoconstriction. Other factors causing arteriolar dilatation include decreased sympathetic activity, increased pCO_2, decreased pH and pO_2, lactic acid, histamine and increased local temperature.

7: CLINICAL CHEMISTRY

1. The following are features of von Gierke's disease:

- ☐ A hyperlipidaemia
- ☐ B autosomal dominant inheritance
- ☐ C hepatosplenomegaly and cardiomegaly in infants
- ☐ D deficiency of glucose-6-phosphate
- ☐ E an association with hypoglycaemia

2. Findings consistent with a diagnosis of untreated phenylketonuria include

- ☐ A eczema
- ☐ B cataracts
- ☐ C an IQ of 100
- ☐ D a reduced blood phenylalanine level
- ☐ E microcephaly

3. An increased cerebrospinal fluid (CSF) globulin:albumin ratio is seen in

- ☐ A multiple sclerosis
- ☐ B acoustic neuroma
- ☐ C neurosyphilis
- ☐ D SLE
- ☐ E encephalitis

4. Thiamine deficiency is associated with

- ☐ A a peripheral neuropathy
- ☐ B an increased incidence in maize eaters
- ☐ C widening of the pulse pressure
- ☐ D reduced blood pyruvate and lactate levels
- ☐ E glossitis

5. A positive 'Clinitest' reaction may occur with

☐ A L-dopa therapy
☐ B salicylate therapy
☐ C alkaptonuria
☐ D galactosaemia
☐ E aminoaciduria

6. Transferrin

☐ A levels are raised by oral contraceptive therapy
☐ B levels are reduced by iron deficiency
☐ C is normally about 70% saturated with iron
☐ D levels are high in haemochromatosis
☐ E is excessively saturated with iron in severe liver disease

7. Elevated serum acid phosphatase is found in

☐ A vitamin D resistant rickets
☐ B Gaucher's disease
☐ C Paget's disease
☐ D carcinoma of the rectum
☐ E Hurler's syndrome

8. The following are major effects of insulin on intermediary metabolism:

☐ A increased uptake of glucose into skeletal muscle
☐ B activation of glycogen synthetase
☐ C insulin deficiency is associated with increased release of free fatty acids
☐ D insulin deficiency is associated with increased protein synthesis
☐ E increased uptake of amino acids

9. Free fatty acids

☐ A inhibit gluconeogenesis
☐ B inhibit glycolysis
☐ C are released from adipose tissue when insulin levels are low
☐ D are released from the adipose tissue during starvation
☐ E stimulate metabolism via the pentose phosphate pathway

10. Abnormal colour of the urine is seen in

☐ A phenylketonuria
☐ B cystinuria
☐ C phenolphthalein therapy
☐ D congenital porphyria
☐ E rifampicin therapy

11. The following may occur in lead poisoning:

☐ A diarrhoea
☐ B abdominal pain relieved by calcium gluconate
☐ C reticulocytosis
☐ D purpura
☐ E peripheral oedema

12. A low serum B12 is associated with

☐ A total gastrectomy
☐ B phenytoin therapy
☐ C pregnancy
☐ D Addisonian pernicious anaemia
☐ E cirrhosis of the liver

13. The following are features of homocystinuria:

☐ A absence of cystathione β-synthetase
☐ B high incidence of renal calculi
☐ C improvement following a high methionine diet
☐ D association with lens dislocation
☐ E association with arterial thrombosis

14. Spontaneous hypoglycaemia occurs in

☐ A thyrotoxicosis
☐ B galactosaemia
☐ C leucine sensitivity
☐ D Addison's disease
☐ E carcinoid syndrome

15. Characteristics of acute intermittent hepatic porphyria include

☐ A motor disturbances
☐ B Mendelian dominant inheritance
☐ C sensory disturbances
☐ D abdominal pain
☐ E hypotension

16. Hypercalcaemia may be caused by

☐ A Addison's disease
☐ B multiple myeloma
☐ C hyperthyroidism
☐ D Paget's disease
☐ E vitamin D intoxication

17. In acute intermittent porphyria

☐ A there is skin photosensitivity
☐ B arthritis may occur
☐ C there is autosomal dominant inheritance
☐ D colicky abdominal pain is a feature
☐ E neurological complications are common

18. Causes of hypoglycaemia include

☐ A acute alcohol toxicity
☐ B hereditary fructose intolerance
☐ C salicylates
☐ D glucagonoma
☐ E falciparum malaria

19. The following statements about iron metabolism are correct:

☐ A most iron is not in the form of haem
☐ B turnover of plasma iron is directly related to haemopoiesis
☐ C take up of iron in marrow is by endocytosis of whole iron-transferrin complexes
☐ D iron absorption is inappropriately high in aplastic anaemia
☐ E plasma iron levels follow a circadian rhythm

20. Hepatic gluconeogenesis may be inhibited by

☐ A alcohol
☐ B glucocorticoids
☐ C glucagon
☐ D insulin
☐ E acidosis

21. Proteinuria of >15–20 g/day is caused by

☐ A amyloidosis
☐ B SLE
☐ C acute renal tubular acidosis
☐ D analgesic nephropathy
☐ E adult Fanconi's syndrome

22. Hypercalcaemia is associated with

☐ A sarcoidosis
☐ B myositis ossificans
☐ C systemic sclerosis
☐ D hypothyroidism
☐ E pulmonary tuberculosis

23. Hypercalciuria occurs in

☐ A nutritional rickets
☐ B ingestion of five pints of milk daily
☐ C sarcoidosis
☐ D renal tubular acidosis
☐ E patients with intestinal hyperabsorption of milk

24. Glucocorticoid hormones

☐ A increase the level of amino acids
☐ B reduce intracellular phosphorus
☐ C increase extracellular potassium
☐ D raise the number of circulating eosinophils
☐ E suppress the production of ACTH

25. Hypoglycaemia occurs after adrenalectomy because of failure of

☐ A gluconeogenesis
☐ B glycogen formation
☐ C glucose absorption from gut
☐ D glycogenolysis
☐ E protein catabolism

26. Haem biosynthesis is abnormal in

☐ A sickle cell trait
☐ B megaloblastic anaemia
☐ C homozygous thalassaemia
☐ D lead poisoning
☐ E acute intermittent porphyria

27. Oxygen uptake by haemoglobin

☐ A increases its buffering capacity
☐ B is increased by 2,3 DPG
☐ C changes iron from the ferrous to ferric form
☐ D is higher in Hb than in HbA
☐ E is increased in the presence of carboxyhaemoglobin

28. Alkaline phosphatase is raised in

☐ A osteoporosis
☐ B osteomalacia
☐ C chronic leukaemia
☐ D post menopause
☐ E Paget's disease

29. The following statements about the Henderson–Hasselbach equation are correct:

☐ A it contains two constants
☐ B the $PaCO_2$ is the partial pressure of CO_2 in arterial blood
☐ C it relates arterial pH, pCO_2 and HCO_3^-
☐ D it relates arterial pH, HCO_3^- and pO_2
☐ E the pKa describes the pH of a buffer at which half the acid molecules are undissociated

30. Magnesium is reduced in

☐ A severe diarrhoea
☐ B chronic dialysis
☐ C acute renal disease
☐ D hyperthyroidism
☐ E idiopathic hypercalcaemia

31. Vitamin D

☐ A is most active in the 25-hydroxycholecalciferol form
☐ B is hydroxylated to 24,25-dihydroxycholecalciferol in the kidney
☐ C the enzyme 1-alpha-hydroxylase catalyses the hydroxylation of 25-HCC in the kidney
☐ D 1,25-hydroxy vitamin D production is stimulated by a high circulating phosphate concentration
☐ E failure of the initial hydroxylation explains the hypocalcaemia of renal failure

32. Chloride depletion

☐ A results in inappropriate acidification of the urine
☐ B results in an inappropriate potassium loss in the kidney
☐ C occurs with chronic respiratory acidosis
☐ D occurs with overtreatment with diuretics
☐ E is associated with hypertriglyceridaemia

33. Hyperuricaemia can be seen in

- ☐ A untreated polycythaemia rubra vera
- ☐ B exfoliative psoriasis
- ☐ C high dose salicylate use
- ☐ D diabetic ketoacidosis
- ☐ E haemophilia

34. The following cause an increase in the concentration of plasma inorganic phosphate:

- ☐ A intravenous infusion of isotonic glucose
- ☐ B delay in separation of plasma from red blood cells
- ☐ C primary hyperparathyroidism
- ☐ D Gram-negative bacterial septicaemia
- ☐ E malignant hyperpyrexia following anaesthesia

ANSWERS AND TEACHING NOTES: CLINICAL CHEMISTRY

1. A E

In von Gierke's disease (type I glycogen storage disease), there is a deficiency of the enzyme glucose-6-phosphatase. It usually presents in infancy, with recurrent hypoglycaemia, hepatomegaly, muscle weakness, cardiac failure (features common to all glycogen storage diseases), in addition to metabolic acidosis, hyperlipidaemia, hyperuricaemia and ketosis. Inheritance is autosomal recessive in common with other 'metabolic-type' disorders.

2. A E

Phenylketonuria is an inborn error of amino acid metabolism. The site of the metabolic block is the phenylalanine hydroxylase pathway. It presents in early childhood with reduced pigmentation, eczema, mental retardation (IQ usually less than 20) and seizures. A raised blood level of phenylalanine is present approximately one week after birth. Early treatment with a low phenylalanine diet is important.

3. A C D

A raised CSF protein is seen with all these conditions, but an increased globulin:albumin ratio due to intrathecal synthesis of immunoglobulin is only seen with multiple sclerosis, neurosyphilis, SLE and cerebral sarcoidosis. Inflammatory diseases, including acoustic neuroma and encephalitis are associated with a low globulin:albumin ratio due to leakage of albumin via the blood–brain barrier.

4. A C

Thiamine (vitamin B_1) deficiency is associated with either 'dry' beri-beri (polyneuritis and weight loss) or 'wet' beri-beri (high output cardiac failure), or Wernicke–Korsakoff syndrome. It occurs in chronic alcoholics and when polished rice is the staple diet. The blood pyruvate level is increased, but there is a decrease in red cell transketolase activity and in excretion of urinary thiamine. Glossitis is a feature of pyridoxine (vitamin B_6) deficiency.

5. A B C D

A positive 'Clinitest' reaction is associated with:

1. Glycosuria e.g. diabetes mellitus, thyrotoxicosis, post-gastrectomy, phaeochromocytoma, severe infection, a lag glucose tolerance curve, and pregnancy (reduced renal threshold).

2. Galactosaemia, hereditary fructosaemia, alkaptonuria.
3. Drugs, e.g. salicylates, isoniazid, L-dopa, vitamin C, tetracyclines.

6. A E

Iron is carried in the plasma, in the Fe^{3+} form, attached to a specific binding protein, transferrin, which is normally about one third saturated with iron. Transferrin levels are raised in iron deficiency anaemia, pregnancy or with oral contraceptives, and with viral hepatitis. Levels are normal or decreased in haemochromatosis.

7. B C

Acid phosphatase is present in the prostate, platelets, red cells and Gaucher's cells. It is raised in carcinoma of the prostate with metastases, following renal examination or passage of a urinary catheter, with Gaucher's disease, metastatic disease with bony involvement, haemolysis and myeloid leukaemia.

8. A B C E

Major effects of insulin are:

Adipose tissue
- Increased glucose entry
- Increased fatty acid synthesis
- Increased lipolysis
- Activation of lipoprotein lipase and hormone-sensitive lipase

Muscle
- Increased glucose uptake
- Increased glycogen synthesis
- Increased amino acid uptake
- Increased protein synthesis
- Decreased protein catabolism

Liver
- Increased glucose uptake
- Increased glycogen synthesis
- Inhibition of gluconeogenesis
- Increased lipogenesis
- Inhibition of ketogenesis

9. B C D

Adipose tissue contains an enzyme, hormone-sensitive lipase (HSL) that hydrolyses triglycerides to produce fatty acids and glycerol. During fasting, when exogenous glucose is unavailable, endogenous adipose tissue triglyceride is converted to free fatty acids and glycerol by lipolysis. Both are transported to the liver where glycerol enters the gluconeogenic pathway. The resultant glucose is released into the blood stream at a time when the plasma glucose would otherwise fall. HSL is inhibited by insulin. Insulin inhibits the release of free fatty acids (FFA) from adipose tissue, therefore a low insulin level is associated with increased release of FFA.

10. C D E

In porphyria, porphyrinogens (δ-amino laevulinic acid (LALA) and prophobilinogen (PBG)) in the urine are colourless, but in ultraviolet light they oxidize to corresponding porphyrins which are dark red. Rifampicin colours urine pink.

11. B C

Clinical features of lead poisoning include intestinal colic, gingivitis, a blue line on the gums, lead encephalopathy and motor neuropathy. Haematological effects include anaemia, basophilic stippling, reticulocytosis and increased serum iron.

12. A D

A low serum B12 is associated with: (i) dietary deficiency (true vegans); (ii) malabsorption due to pernicious anaemia, partial/total gastrectomy or Crohn's disease, ileal resection, blind loop syndrome or fish tapeworm.

13. A D E

Homocystinuria is due to a metabolic block (deficiency of cystathione β-synthetase) in the conversion of homocystine and serine to cystathionine. It is characterized by mental retardation, seizures, spastic paraplegia, osteoporosis, cataracts, thromboembolic disease, downwards dislocation of the lens, arachnodactyly and high arched palate. Plasma methionine and urinary homocystine are elevated. Treatment is by dietary restriction of methionine with cystine supplementation.

14. B C D

Spontaneous hypoglycaemia occurs in glycogen storage diseases (types I and III), galactosaemia, fructose intolerance, leucine sensitivity, Addison's disease and hypopituitarism, post-gastrectomy syndrome, beta-cell islet tumours, alcoholic cirrhosis and hypothyroidism.

15. A B C D

Clinical features of acute intermittent porphyria include:

fragile skin
GI – abdominal pain, vomiting and constipation
CNS – peripheral neuropathy, confusion and psychosis
Cardiovascular – tachycardia and hypertension.

16. A B C E

Hypercalcaemia may result from (i) increased intake/absorption, e.g. vitamin D excess, sarcoidosis, IV therapy; (ii) increased bone resorption, e.g. malignancy, hyperparathyroidism, thyrotoxicosis, immobilization, renal failure; (iii) increased renal reabsorption, e.g. thiazide diuretic therapy; (iv) miscellaneous, e.g. Addison's disease, acromegaly, vitamin D intoxication, tuberculosis, phaeochromocytoma.

17. C D E

See answer to Question 15.

18. A B C E

See answer to Question 14.

19. B C E

Approximately 60–70% of total body iron is in haem form. Iron absorption is increased by marrow erythropoietic activity, and is therefore low in aplastic anaemia.

20. D

Hepatic gluconeogenesis is stimulated by glucagon, adrenaline and cortisol and inhibited by insulin.

21. A B

Massive proteinuria is associated with the nephrotic syndrome which may be secondary to diabetes mellitus, SLE, inferior vena cava or renal vein thrombosis, amyloidosis, or malaria due to *P. malariae*.

22. A

See answer to Question 16.

23. B C D

Hypercalciuria occurs in the presence of both hypercalcaemia and normocalcaemia.

Hypercalcaemia

- increased bone resorption (primary hypoparathyroidism, malignancy, multiple myeloma, immobilization and hyperthyroidism)
- increased gut absorption (vitamin D excess and sarcoidosis)

Normocalcaemia

- increased bone resorption (list as above plus osteoporosis, renal tubular acidosis and Paget's disease)
- increased gut absorption (list as above and idiopathic hypercalciuria).

24. A B E

Actions of glucocorticoids include:

(i) Glycogenesis (liver)
(ii) Gluconeogenesis from protein (liver)
(iii) Increased protein catabolism
(iv) Lipolysis, increased free fatty acid mobilization, oxidation and increased ketone production
(v) Increased plasma glucose
(vi) Anti-inflammatory and anti-allergic properties
(vii) Increased resistance to stress
(viii) Decreased lymphocytes and eosinophils; increased neutrophils, platelets and red cells
(ix) Increased urinary calcium
(x) Increased secretion of hydrochloric acid and pepsin

25. A

The important effects of adrenalectomy are a fall in plasma potassium, and hypoglycaemia through inhibition of gluconeogenesis. Plasma volume is reduced, resulting in hypotension and shock.

26. D E

In acute intermittent porphyria there is a defect in the conversion of porphobilinogen to uroporphyrinogen. Lead poisoning also inhibits several enzymes in haem synthesis. Thalassaemias and sickle cell disease are disorders of globin synthesis.

27. A C D

2,3-DPG binds haemoglobin, stabilizing the deoxy form, and reduces the affinity of haemoglobin for oxygen, causing the release of oxygen. Oxygen binds to the ferrous form in haem to form oxyhaemoglobin, where the haem group is in the ferric form. The oxygen affinity is increased in cells containing fetal haemoglobin and with methaemoglobin and carboxyhaemoglobin, leading to tissue hypoxia.

28. B E

Alkaline phosphatase is raised in: growing children, pregnancy, bone disease (e.g. metastatic malignancy, Paget's disease, osteomalacia, hyperparathyroidism) and liver disease (e.g. obstructive jaundice, cirrhosis, malignancy, space-occupying lesions).

29. A C E

The Henderson–Hasselbach equation describes the relationship of arterial pH to $PaCO_2$, bicarbonate and two constants.

$$pH = 6.1 + \log \frac{[HCO_3^-]}{0.235 \times [PaCO_2]}$$

where $PaCO_2$ is the partial pressure of CO_2 in alveolar air (kPa).

30. A B

Causes of magnesium deficiency include: chronic alcoholism, severe diarrhoea, malabsorption and fistulae, diuretic therapy, chronic dialysis, acute pancreatitis.

31. B C

Cholecalciferol (vitamin D3) is hydroxylated first in the liver to produce 25-HCC and next in the kidney to generate both 1,25-HCC and 24,25-DHCC. 25-hydroxycholecalciferol is the main circulating form of the vitamin. Further hydroxylation is necessary to confer biological activity. Production of 1,25-DHCC is stimulated by a low circulating phosphate concentration, a high circulating parathyroid hormone (PTH), oestrogen, prolactin and growth hormone.

32. A C D

Hypochloraemic alkalosis may occur with vomiting and diarrhoea, over treatment with diuretics, chronic respiratory acidosis, diabetic acidosis and Addison's disease. Metabolic effects of prolonged vomiting include hypochloraemic alkalosis, paradoxical aciduria, compensatory hypoventilation, and inhibition of renal HCO_3^- excretion.

33. A B D

Causes of hyperuricaemia:

(i) Increased purine synthesis e.g. primary gout, Lesch–Nyhan syndrome.
(ii) Increased purine turnover e.g. myeloproliferative and lymphoproliferative disorders, polycythaemia, severe exfoliative psoriasis.
(iii) Decreased excretion of uric acid e.g. primary gout, renal failure, diabetic ketoacidosis.
(iv) Drugs e.g. thiazide and loop diuretics, pyrazinamide, salicylate in low doses, cytotoxic agents and alcohol.

34. B E

During carbohydrate utilization, phosphate and potassium enter the cells with glucose. Intravenous glucose infusion may cause severe hypophosphataemia, therefore blood for measurement of inorganic phosphate should be taken from fasting patients. If rapid separation of plasma from red blood cells is not achieved, erythrocyte phosphates and inorganic phosphates will cause a false high concentration of serum phosphates. Parathyroid hormone causes phosphaturia and a reduced serum concentration of inorganic phosphate. Gram-negative septicaemia causes hypophosphataemia.

Malignant hyperpyrexia
↑ temp
acidosis (↑ PO_4^{2-})

NB PO_4^{2-} [illegible] to Ca^{2+}

1. The following statements are true:

- ☐ A logarithmic scales measure percentage changes in a variable
- ☐ B a log-normal distribution is a skew distribution
- ☐ C in distributions which are markedly skewed, the arithmetic mean is a more appropriate measure than the geometric mean
- ☐ D the mode is the value that occurs most frequently
- ☐ E in a positively skewed distribution, the median is greater than the mode, but less than the mean

2. The following statements are true:

- ☐ A the standard error of the mean (SEM) is generally smaller than the standard deviation
- ☐ B the standard error of the mean provides a measure of the spread of observations around the mean
- ☐ C $SD = \frac{SEM}{\sqrt{n}}$
- ☐ D the mean and standard deviation of a random sample will generally be different from the mean and standard of the population
- ☐ E the coefficient of variation is derived from the range

3. In a hypertension screening programme among 1550 males aged 30–69 years, both the mean and median of the diastolic blood pressure distribution are approximately 83 mmHg and the standard deviation 12 mmHg. The following statements are true:

- ☐ A approximately 95% of the men have diastolic blood pressures between 59–107 mmHg
- ☐ B the distribution is nearly symmetrical
- ☐ C 99% of the observations lie within 2.6 SE of the mean
- ☐ D the range 59–107 mmHg will include the mean of all screened males with a 95% probability
- ☐ E 5% of the men will have a diastolic blood pressure greater than 107 mmHg

4. The following statements about the chi-squared test are true:

☐ A it is used as an alternative to the *t*-test to determine the difference between two means
☐ B it is used to test the difference between frequencies
☐ C the greater the value of the chi-squared test, the less likely it is to be significant
☐ D the number of degrees of freedom is the number of independent comparisons
☐ E the null hypothesis is applied

5. The correlation coefficient *(r)* between two variables is estimated from a sample of pairs of observations. The following statements are true:

☐ A if $r = 0.1$, there is unlikely to be a significant relationship between the two variables
☐ B if $r = 0.3$ with $p < 0.005$, then there is no significant correlation between the two variables
☐ C r may be positive or negative
☐ D if $r = 0.9$, there is a good negative correlation between the two variables
☐ E the observed result with a probability of 0.02 is more significant than with a probability of 0.05

6. In a preliminary trial, a new oral hypoglycaemic is administered to 12 diabetic patients

☐ A the statistical significance of the fall in blood glucose may be analysed by Student's paired *t*-test
☐ B unlike Student's *t*-test, non-parametric tests can be used on data which have a skew distribution
☐ C a fall in blood glucose with a probability value of $p > 0.05$ would indicate significant effect of the drug
☐ D one in 20 such studies would be expected to show a significant effect of the hypoglycaemic agents on blood glucose by chance alone
☐ E use of double blind methods means that neither the doctor nor the patients would be aware whether the drug or a placebo was being given

7. The following statements about retrospective and prospective studies are true:

☐ A in a prospective study the cohort originally selected consists of persons who are found to have the disease
☐ B a retrospective study involves a survey of the prevalence of the disease in different strata of the population
☐ C prospective studies allow direct determination of incidence rates
☐ D the retrospective approach has the advantage that there is little or no bias in the assessment of exposure to the suspected factor
☐ E the prospective approach may be used to study the aetiology of a rare disease

8. The table below shows the results from a screening test for diabetes used on 10,000 persons (Test A). The cut-off level used was 8 mmol/l or above of glucose

Results from a screening test for diabetes

Screening test results	*True Diagnosis*		
	Diabetic	*Non-diabetic*	*Total*
Positive	34	20	54
Negative	116	9,830	9,946
Total	150	9,850	10,000

In Test B, the screening cut-off level was lowered to 6 mmol/l or above of blood glucose

☐ A sensitivity of Test A = 22.6%
☐ B specificity of Test A = 75%
☐ C the specificity of Test A is greater than that of Test B
☐ D the number of false positives is greater with Test A than Test B
☐ E initial screening provides a prevalence estimate and subsequent screenings, an incidence estimate

9. The following statements are true:

- ☐ A in a normal distribution the mean, mode and median coincide
- ☐ B the mode is the most frequently occurring value
- ☐ C the median has an equal number of values above and below it
- ☐ D the mode is the maximum point on a frequency distribution curve
- ☐ E about 95% of observations lie within two standard deviations of the mean

10. The following statements are true:

- ☐ A standard deviation gives a measure of the spread of values above and below it
- ☐ B the range is the difference between the highest and lowest values
- ☐ C standard deviation is the square of the variance of the group
- ☐ D about 68% of observations lie within one standard deviation of the mean
- ☐ E 99% of observations lie within 2.6 standard variations of the mean

11. In a study of 100 AIDS patients, the distribution of time from AIDS diagnosis to death was positively skewed, with a peak at 2 years and a median survival of 3 years. The following statements are correct:

- ☐ A 50% of patients were dead by three years
- ☐ B the mean survival will be less than the median survival
- ☐ C most patients died earlier rather than later
- ☐ D the mean survival is the best guide to the average length of life
- ☐ E the mean survival is greater than three years

12. In a study of patients with seizures, 50 patients had EEGs performed, of which 30 had abnormalities. Ten per cent of normal people have EEG abnormalities. The following statements are true:

- ☐ A the specificity is 62%
- ☐ B the specificity is 5%
- ☐ C the value of the EEG in detecting seizures depends upon the prevalence of seizures
- ☐ D the positive predictive value is 75%
- ☐ E if the prevalence of seizures in the population is 5%, and 1000 persons are screened in a month, the number of false positives will be 30

13. A normal population distribution is required for the following statistical tests:

- ☐ A Student's *t*-test
- ☐ B chi-squared
- ☐ C standard error of the mean
- ☐ D variance estimation
- ☐ E Spearman's rank coefficient

14. Two variables, X and Y, are studied for a population and the simple correlation coefficient (*r*) is equal to + 0.8. The correlation coefficient indicates that

- ☐ A variable X and variable Y have the same unit of measure
- ☐ B variable X and variable Y are causally related
- ☐ C there is an inverse linear relationship between variable X and variable Y
- ☐ D variable X and variable Y are strongly associated
- ☐ E a unit increase in variable X is associated with a corresponding increase by 0.8 in variable Y

15. The prevalence rate of a disease has the following characteristics:

- ☐ A it measures all of the current cases in the community
- ☐ B it is dependent on the duration of illness
- ☐ C it is dependent on the incidence of disease
- ☐ D it can be used to determine the health needs of a community
- ☐ E it can be estimated from a cross-sectional study

16. True statements concerning Type I error include

- ☐ A it is the rejection of a null hypothesis that is actually true
- ☐ B it is often assigned a value of 0.05 in studies
- ☐ C it is also called the alpha error
- ☐ D it is used to help determine an appropriate sample size for a study
- ☐ E it is equal to one minus the beta error

17. The standard error of the mean of a sample is

- ☐ A derived from the standard deviation of the sample
- ☐ B based on a normal distribution
- ☐ C used to determine confidence limits
- ☐ D increased as the sample size increases
- ☐ E halved if the sample size is quadrupled

18. The following rates are correctly matched with the appropriate application:

- ☐ A crude rate – is a summary rate for the entire population
- ☐ B direct age-adjusted rate – uses a standard population
- ☐ C indirect age-adjusted rate – is a fictitious rate
- ☐ D incidence rate – is used as an attack rate in epidemic investigations
- ☐ E age-specific rate – can be compared in different populations

19. The weaknesses of retrospective studies of the role of a suspected factor in the aetiology of a disease, as compared with prospective studies, are that

- ☐ A they are more costly and take longer
- ☐ B there may be bias in determining the presence or absence of a suspected factor
- ☐ C there may be bias in determining the presence or absence of the resulting disease
- ☐ D it is more difficult to obtain controls
- ☐ E it is more difficult to assure comparability of cases and controls

20. Controls are needed in a case-control retrospective study because

- ☐ A they are matched to the cases for suspected aetiological factors
- ☐ B they may be followed to determine if they develop the disease in question
- ☐ C they increase the sample size, so that statistical significance may be achieved
- ☐ D they allow evaluation of whether or not the frequency of a characteristic or past exposure among the cases is different from that among comparable persons in the population who are free of the disease
- ☐ E they allow a comparison of disease rates across study groups

21. To be causally related to a disease an aetiological factor must satisfy the following conditions:

- ☐ A the factor is found more frequently among the diseased than non-diseased
- ☐ B exposure to the factor must precede the development of the disease
- ☐ C elimination of the factor reduces the risk of the disease
- ☐ D the factor is found among all cases with the disease
- ☐ E the factor is not found among any persons without the disease

ANSWERS AND TEACHING NOTES: STATISTICS AND EPIDEMIOLOGY

1. **A B D E**

   On an arithmetic scale, equal distances measure equal absolute distances, while on a logarithmic scale, equal distances measure equal proportional differences (i.e. percentage change in a variable). A log–normal distribution is a skewed distribution when graphed using an arithmetic scale, but is a normal distribution when graphed using a logarithmic scale. The geometric mean is used as a substitute for the arithmetic mean when the distribution is skewed. The mode is the most commonly occurring value in a series of values. It is useful in practical epidemiological work, such as for determining the peak disease occurrence in the investigation of a disease outbreak.

2. **A D**

   The standard error measures the variability of a sample statistic (i.e. mean or proportion) in relation to the true population characteristic (i.e how accurate is the sample mean as an estimate of the population mean?). The standard deviation is the measure of the variability of the observations:

   $$\text{Standard error} = \frac{\text{Standard deviation of observations in a sample}}{\sqrt{\text{Sample size}}}$$

   $$\text{The coefficient of variation (\%)} = \frac{\text{SD}}{\text{Mean}} \times 100$$

3. **A B D**

   The distribution of diastolic blood pressure is normal or Gaussian, because the mean and median values are equal. Therefore, 95% of observations fall within two standard deviations (SD) (not standard errors, SE) from the mean or between 59 and 107 mmHg. 2.5% of the men will have a diastolic blood pressure greater than 107 mmHg.

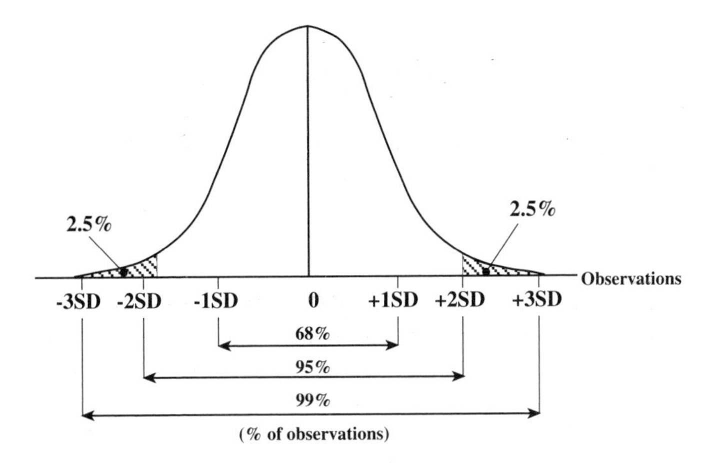

4. **B D E**

The chi-squared test is used to determine the difference between observed and expected frequencies or between two or more frequencies. The calculated χ^2 value is compared with a critical value of χ^2 from tables, at a predetermined significance level and appropriate degrees of freedom. The larger the χ^2 value the smaller the probability *p*, and the more likely it is that the null hypothesis is untrue.

5. **A C E**

The correlation coefficient (*r*) describes the strength of the linear relationship between two variables. Its value can range from –1 (high negative correlation) to +1 (high positive correlation).

Correlation coefficient (r)	*Degree of association*
0.8 to 1.0	Strong
0.5 to 0.8	Moderate
0.2 to 0.5	Weak
0 to 0.2	Negligible

r may be strong but statistically insignificant because of a small sample size.

6. A B D E

A paired *t*-test could be used to compare the means of the blood glucose in the 12 diabetic patients before and after administration of the new oral hypoglycaemic drug. Non-parametric tests are used when the data are not normally distributed or when data are qualitative. Examples of non-parametric tests include: chi-squared (χ^2) test, Wilcoxon rank sum test, Mann Whitney U test, and Wilcoxon signed rank test.

7. C

In a prospective cohort study, exposed and non-exposed populations are identified and followed over time to determine the incidence of a specific clinical disease or event, e.g. a population of smokers and non-smokers are followed to provide comparison rates for lung cancer or heart disease. Cross-sectional studies provide information on disease prevalence in a population. Case-control (retrospective studies) compare persons with and without a disease to determine possible associations or risk factors for the disease in question. Bias may influence the recall of exposure in these studies if possible associations are known, such as the association between cigarette smoking and lung cancer. A case-control study is relatively easy and inexpensive to conduct, since long term follow up is not required, and is therefore suitable for rare diseases.

8. A C E

The sensitivity of a screening test is the test's ability to identify correctly those individuals who truly have diabetes.

$$= \frac{a}{a + c} \times 100 = \frac{34}{150} = 22.67\%$$

The specificity is the test's ability to identify correctly those individuals who do not have the disease.

$$= \frac{d}{b + d} \times 100 = \frac{9830}{9850} = 99.80\%$$

Lowering the screening cut-off level increases the sensitivity and number of false positives and decreases the specificity and number of false negatives. The first time that screening is carried out is called the 'prevalence screen', since cases of diabetes will have been present for varying lengths of time. During the second round of screening, most cases will have had their onset between the first and second screening. Therefore second, and subsequent screenings are called 'incidence screens'.

9. **A B C D E**
The mode is the most frequently observed value in a series of values and is therefore the maximum point in a frequency distribution curve. The median is the central value of a series of observations arranged in order of magnitude.

10. **A B D E**
The standard deviation is the square root of the variance. In a normal distribution, approximately 68% of the observations fall within one standard variation of the mean; and 99% fall within 2.6 standard deviations from the mean.

11. **A C E**
In a positively skewed distribution, the mean will be greater than the median, which in turn is greater than the mode.

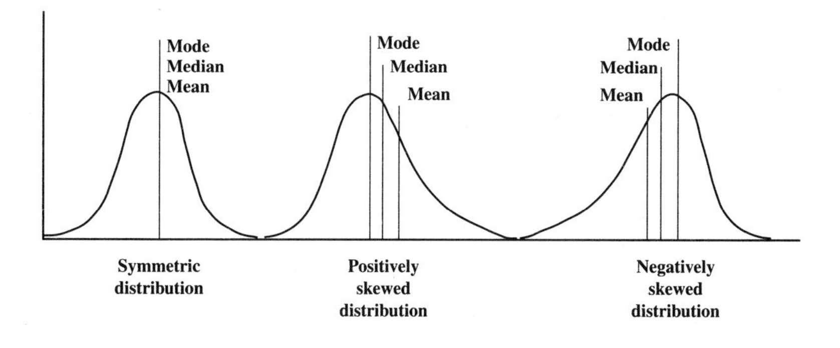

12. E

EEG test result	*True diagnosis*	
	Seizures	*No seizures*
Positive	30	10
Negative	20	90
Total	50	100

Sensitivity = 30/50 x 100 = 60%; Specificity = 90/100 x 100 = 90%

The sensitivity and specificity are independent of the disease prevalence in the population being tested. The low sensitivity of EEG implies an unacceptably high false negative rate for a serious condition such as seizures.

The positive predictive value is a test's ability to identify those persons who truly have the disease from among all those persons whose screening tests are positive. In this example the positive predictive value (75%) is the number of persons with disease who screen positive (30) divided by the total number of persons who screen positive (40).

Out of 1000 people screened, 50 will have the disease, a prevalence of 5%. Now a + c = 50, with a sensitivity of 60%, means that a = 30 and c = 20 (false negative). Now b +d = 950 with a specificity of 90%, thus d = 855 and b (false positive) = 95.

EEG test results	*True diagnosis*		
	Seizures	*No seizures*	*Total*
Positive	30	95	125
Negative	20	855	875
Total	50	950	1000

13. C D

Non-parametric tests make no assumptions about the underlying distribution of the sample. Parametric tests assume that the populations from which samples are taken should be normally distributed, and the variances of the samples are the same. Spearman's and Kendall's rank correlation coefficients are the non-parametric alternatives to Pearson's correlation coefficient.

14. D

The correlation coefficient is used to indicate the extent that two variables change with one another in a linear manner. The two variables can have the same or different units of measure, but the correlation coefficient is unitless. A –1 value indicates a strong inverse linear association (an increase in one variable is associated with a decrease in the other) while +1 indicates a strong direct linear association. Causality cannot be determined from the correlation coefficient, because the two variables may be associated through a third variable rather than directly.

15. A B C D E

The prevalence rate is the number of current cases (old and new) of a specified disease during a specified time period divided by the estimated mid-interval population at risk. Since the prevalence rate includes all cases in the community, it is determined by both the incidence and the duration of the disease process. It can also be used to determine the health needs of the community since it measures the total illness within the community.

16. A B C D

The type I error, or alpha error, is the rejection of a null hypothesis that is actually true. Type I error is used to help determine the sample size of a study and to test the null hypothesis, which is often rejected at the arbitrary cut off of 5% probability due to chance. The beta error is the acceptance as true of a false null hypothesis, and the formula 1 minus the beta error is used to calculate the power of the study.

17. A B C E

The standard error of the mean is an estimate of the standard deviation of the population, based on the standard deviation of a sample. The standard error of the mean is equal to the standard deviation of the sample divided by the square root of the sample size; therefore the standard error of the mean decreases as the sample size increases. The standard error of the mean is based on the fact that the means of the samples follow a normal distribution, even if the samples do not. The standard error of the mean is used to determine confidence limits.

18. A B C D E

Crude rates are summary rates for an entire population. They are easy to calculate because only the number of events and the total population are needed. They cannot, however, be used to compare events in different populations because the rate is dependent on the age–sex composition of the total population.

Adjusted rates are summary rates for the total population, but they are fictitious. By using a standard population or standard age-specific rates, they equalize the differences in the population at risk so that the rates are comparable. Adjusted rates are difficult to calculate because the demographic composition of the population must be known. They are frequently used to compare birth and death rates in different populations and for international comparisons because they take into consideration the age composition of the different populations. They are seldom used for epidemic investigations of acute diseases

Age-specific rates are calculated for various segments of the population. Although they are difficult to calculate because more information about the demographic composition of the community must be known than with other rates, they can be used to compare events in similar age groups in different populations.

Attack rates are a form of incidence rate – that is, the number of new cases of a specified disease during a specific time interval divided by the total population at risk during the same time interval. They are used in epidemic investigations using a particular population, which is observed for a limited period of time.

19. B

Although time consuming, a cohort study allows for determination of a population-based rate of the event under question. A case-control study, on the other hand, is relatively easy and inexpensive to conduct since long term follow-up is not required. In a cohort study, potential bias is lessened because exposure can be determined prior to the onset of disease, whereas with a case control study, there is potential for bias in the selection of subjects since a case control study is not population based. The incidence rate of an event or disease for exposed and non-exposed populations can be calculated for a cohort study but not in a case-control study. Causality cannot be determined for either a case-control or a cohort study.

20. D

See explanation to Question 19.

21. A B C

Causation is defined by various criteria in addition to risk assessment. These include biological plausibility, appropriate temporal relationships between exposure and disease or event, consistent outcomes, and observations across several studies, dose-response relationships, and finally an experimental or animal study confirmation or association.

1. The following drugs are contraindicated during breast feeding:

☐ A warfarin
☐ B propylthiouracil
☐ C lithium
☐ D gold salts
☐ E insulin

2. Aminoglycoside antibiotics

☐ A are metabolized extensively by the liver
☐ B are more ototoxic when combined with a loop diuretic
☐ C accumulate in tissues as treatment progresses
☐ D do not effectively treat *Streptococcus faecalis* infections
☐ E are nephrotoxic

3. The following drugs are known to be teratogenic in man:

☐ A methyldopa
☐ B enalapril
☐ C warfarin
☐ D carbamazepine
☐ E paracetamol

4. The total daily dose of the following drugs should be reduced in patients who have a glomerular filtration rate of less than 30 ml/min:

☐ A erythromycin
☐ B metronidazole
☐ C ciprofloxacin
☐ D enalapril
☐ E frusemide

5. Treatment with the following drugs is recognized as a cause of constipation:

☐ A cholestyramine
☐ B antacids containing magnesium
☐ C disopyramide
☐ D verapamil
☐ E tricyclic antidepressants

6. Treatment with the following drugs is a recognized cause of hyponatraemia:

☐ A carbamazepine
☐ B lithium
☐ C frusemide
☐ D desmopressin
☐ E acyclovir

7. Hepatic first pass metabolism is clinically significant for the following drugs:

☐ A enalapril
☐ B propranolol
☐ C isosorbide dinitrate
☐ D cholestyramine
☐ E ethinyl oestradiol

8. The following may enhance or prolong the hypoglycaemic effect of sulphonylureas:

☐ A acute alcohol intoxication
☐ B co-trimoxazole
☐ C lithium
☐ D bendrofluazide
☐ E rifampicin

9. The following are recognized causes of a raised fasting serum triglyceride concentration:

- ☐ A high ethanol intake
- ☐ B treatment with propranolol
- ☐ C treatment with nifedipine
- ☐ D chronic renal failure
- ☐ E treatment with cholestyramine

10. Zidovudine

- ☐ A blocks viral ribonucleic acid (RNA) synthesis
- ☐ B must be given by prolonged IV injection
- ☐ C is contraindicated in patients with severe neutropenia
- ☐ D has a prolonged half-life of several days
- ☐ E is a recognized cause of nail pigmentation

11. Patients with acute intermittent porphyria should avoid

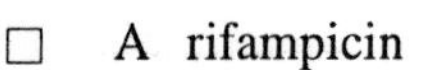

- ☐ A rifampicin
- ☐ B aspirin
- ☐ C phenytoin
- ☐ D chlorpromazine
- ☐ E chlorpropamide

12. Aspirin potentiates the action of the following:

- ☐ A tetracycline
- ☐ B chlorpropamide
- ☐ C benzodiazepines
- ☐ D warfarin
- ☐ E sulphonamides

13. Nephrotoxicity is described with the following drugs:

☐ A gentamicin
☐ B rifampicin
☐ C oxytetracycline
☐ D ampicillin
☐ E erythromycin

14. The following should be avoided in patients on monoamine oxidase inhibitor therapy:

☐ A phentolamine
☐ B imipramine
☐ C sulphonamide
☐ D coffee
☐ E pethidine

15. Photosensitivity is a recognized complication of treatment with

☐ A chlorpromazine
☐ B tetracyclines
☐ C aspirin
☐ D chloroquine
☐ E oral hypoglycaemic agents

16. The simultaneous administration of the following pairs of drugs is potentially hazardous:

☐ A oral contraceptives and rifampicin
☐ B warfarin and chloral hydrate
☐ C digoxin and erythromycin
☐ D L-dopa and phenelzine
☐ E digoxin and propranolol

17. Intrahepatic cholestatic jaundice occurs with

☐ A norethandrolone
☐ B carbon tetrachloride
☐ C halothane
☐ D isoniazid
☐ E amitriptyline

18. The following are features of treatment with phenytoin:

☐ A after a steady state is reached, doubling the dose will approximately double the new steady state plasma concentration
☐ B a loading dose is needed to achieve a rapid effect
☐ C toxicity is associated with a gastrointestinal haemorrhage
☐ D toxicity is associated with a macrocytic anaemia
☐ E protein bound iodine is decreased

19. Measurement of drug concentration in plasma is useful for monitoring

☐ A anticoagulant therapy
☐ B lithium
☐ C tricyclic antidepressants
☐ D tobramycin
☐ E drugs with a small toxic:therapeutic ratio

20. There is evidence that the following drugs are teratogenic:

☐ A aspirin
☐ B sulphonylureas
☐ C phenytoin
☐ D cortisone
☐ E Fansidar

21. Specific therapy (in addition to general support) is often indicated in poisoning by

- ☐ A ferrous sulphate
- ☐ B paracetamol
- ☐ C tricyclic antidepressants
- ☐ D morphine
- ☐ E cyanide

22. Digoxin toxicity may be enhanced by

- ☐ A thyrotoxic heart failure
- ☐ B prolonged use of thiazide diuretics
- ☐ C hypercalcaemia
- ☐ D propranolol
- ☐ E left ventricular failure

23. Gynaecomastia is a recognized side effect of

- ☐ A digoxin
- ☐ B spironolactone
- ☐ C propranolol
- ☐ D methysergide
- ☐ E stilboestrol

24. Galactorrhoea is a recognized side effect of

- ☐ A methyldopa
- ☐ B haloperidol
- ☐ C phenothiazine
- ☐ D spironolactone
- ☐ E imipramine

25. Ergotamine

- ☐ A is a powerful vasoconstrictor
- ☐ B is an alpha-adrenoreceptor blocker
- ☐ C is useful in the treatment of migraine
- ☐ D causes post-partum contraction of the uterus
- ☐ E is chemically related to methysergide

26. The following drugs should not be used or require dose adjustment in renal failure:

- ☐ A nitrofurantoin
- ☐ B diazepam
- ☐ C chlorpropamide
- ☐ D amphotericin
- ☐ E magnesium trisilicate mixture

27. The benefits of dopamine therapy (< 5 μg/kg/min) in cardiogenic shock include

- ☐ A a rise in diastolic blood pressure
- ☐ B arteriolar constriction
- ☐ C slowing of the heart
- ☐ D vasodilation of the renal vasculature
- ☐ E increased force of cardiac contraction

28. An increased heart rate is characteristically caused by

- ☐ A glyceryl trinitrate
- ☐ B sotalol
- ☐ C digitoxin
- ☐ D isoprenaline
- ☐ E pethidine

29. The following drugs are directly hepatotoxic:

- ☐ A methotrexate
- ☐ B colchicine
- ☐ C azathioprine
- ☐ D neomycin
- ☐ E 6-mercaptopurine

30. Peripheral neuropathy may occur with the following drugs:

- ☐ A vinblastine
- ☐ B vincristine
- ☐ C nitrofurantoin
- ☐ D isoniazid
- ☐ E rifampicin

31. Pulmonary fibrosis may be caused by

- ☐ A methysergide
- ☐ B busulphan
- ☐ C ethacrynic acid
- ☐ D penicillins
- ☐ E cyclophosphamide

32. Aplastic anaemia can occur with the following drug therapy:

- ☐ A pyrimethamine
- ☐ B propranolol
- ☐ C sulphonamides
- ☐ D gold
- ☐ E aspirin

33. Erythema nodosum may be caused by

☐ A sulphonamides
☐ B penicillin
☐ C phenobarbitone
☐ D paracetamol
☐ E dapsone

34. Treatment with gold salts may produce

☐ A nephrotoxicity
☐ B diarrhoea
☐ C skin pigmentation
☐ D gout
☐ E aplastic anaemia

35. Recognized complications of phenytoin therapy include

☐ A ataxia
☐ B megaloblastic anaemia
☐ C osteomalacia
☐ D hypocalcaemia
☐ E gum hypertrophy

36. Recognized acute hypersensitivity reactions occurring with heparin therapy include

☐ A alopecia
☐ B urticaria
☐ C hyperkalaemia
☐ D muscle pain
☐ E rhinitis

37. In individuals with G6PDH deficiency the following may cause a haemolytic anaemia:

- ☐ A nitrofurantoin
- ☐ B phenacetin
- ☐ C sulphonamides
- ☐ D dapsone
- ☐ E primaquine

38. Raynaud's phenomenon may be caused by

- ☐ A ergotamine
- ☐ B propranolol
- ☐ C phenothiazine
- ☐ D salicylates
- ☐ E clonidine

39. The following may cause hyperuricaemia:

- ☐ A pyrazinamide
- ☐ B zidovudine
- ☐ C frusemide
- ☐ D hydrochlorothiazide
- ☐ E high dose aspirin

40. The following drugs require reduced dosage with severe renal impairment:

- ☐ A gentamicin
- ☐ B NSAIDs
- ☐ C ranitidine
- ☐ D erythromycin
- ☐ E rifampicin

41. In poisoning

- ☐ A ethylene glycol leads to metabolic acidosis
- ☐ B aminophylline leads to hyperkalaemia
- ☐ C N-acetyl cysteine improves mortality in hepatic encephalopathy caused by paracetamol overdose
- ☐ D charcoal haemoperfusion increases elimination of phenobarbitone
- ☐ E quinine may lead to blindness

42. Breakthrough bleeding or pregnancy may occur in a woman on the combined oral contraceptive pill and the following drugs:

- ☐ A cimetidine
- ☐ B rifampicin
- ☐ C phenytoin
- ☐ D carbamazepine
- ☐ E indomethacin

43. The following drugs and adverse effects are correctly paired:

- ☐ A doxorubicin and cardiomyopathy
- ☐ B methotrexate and mouth ulcers/mucositis
- ☐ C busulphan and pulmonary fibrosis
- ☐ D vincristine and thrombocytopenia
- ☐ E cyclophosphamide and haemorrhagic cystitis

44. Light sensitivity may be an adverse effect of the following drugs:

- ☐ A aspirin
- ☐ B penicillin
- ☐ C chlorpropamide
- ☐ D nalidixic acid
- ☐ E griseofulvin

45. Sodium valproate

☐ A can cause rapid weight gain
☐ B can cause fatal hepatotoxicity
☐ C induces liver enzymes
☐ D can cause tremor
☐ E anticonvulsant effect is related linearly to the plasma concentration

46. Interferon-alfa

☐ A is a non-natural synthetic antiviral agent
☐ B enhances the expression of the major histocompatibility complex antigens
☐ C suppresses viral replication
☐ D has shown some anti-tumour effect in certain solid tumours
☐ E has dose-related side effects

47. Recognized side effects of thiazides include

☐ A hypercholesterolaemia
☐ B hypochloraemia
☐ C impotence
☐ D agranulocytosis
☐ E peripheral neuropathy

ANSWERS AND TEACHING NOTES: PHARMACOLOGY

1. **C D**

   Maternal treatment with lithium can lead to tremor and involuntary movements in the neonate. Gold salts cause renal and haematological toxicity in neonates. Insulin-dependent diabetics are encouraged to breast feed.

2. **B C E**

   Aminoglycosides are cleared almost completely by renal excretion. Frusemide is also directly ototoxic. When co-administration of an aminoglycoside and a loop diuretic is required, bumetamide is preferred as it is less ototoxic. There is gradual tissue accumulation of aminoglycoside antibiotics even when serum levels are still within normal limits. For this reason toxicity is more likely after one week of treatment. Adverse effects are less likely if the peak serum concentration of gentamicin is less than 10 μg/ml and the trough is less than 2 μg/ml.

3. **B C D**

   Hypertensive pregnant women may be treated safely with methyldopa, but all angiotensin-converting enzyme inhibitors should be avoided in pregnancy. Warfarin may cause abnormalities of fetal cartilage and bone and, rarely, aplasia. Birth defects are present in 7% of babies born to mothers taking anti-convulsant drugs. Carbamazepine can cause craniofacial defects and finger nail hypoplasia.

4. **C D**

   The main excretion route for erythromycin is via the liver. Metronidazole is excreted via the liver and gastrointestinal tract. Ciprofloxacin and enalapril are excreted by the kidney. There is significant renal excretion of frusemide, and it is necessary to increase the dose in renal failure.

5. **A C D E**

   Cholestyramine may also be used to treat diarrhoea associated with bile salt malabsorption. Antacids containing calcium carbonate or aluminium hydroxide cause constipation, but magnesium salts cause diarrhoea. Disopyramide and tricyclic antidepressants have anticholinergic side effects.

6. **A C D**
   The mechanism for the development of hyponatraemia with carbamazepine is uncertain, but it probably involves modulation of the effect of arginine vasopressin. Lithium may cause nephrogenic diabetes insipidus and thus hypernatraemia. Desmopressin is an arginine vasopressin analogue and causes retention of free water.

7. **A B C E**
   Enalapril is metabolized to the active compound, enalaprilat. Isosorbide dinitrate is metabolized to the mononitrate, which if taken orally provides more predictable blood levels. Cholestyramine is a resin which is not absorbed. The relatively high doses of ethinyl oestradiol to which the liver is exposed in order to deliver adequate concentrations may be responsible for some of the adverse effects of oestrogen therapy.

8. **A B**
   Alcohol inhibits gluconeogenesis and may precipitate hypoglycaemia in patients treated with sulphonylureas. Sulphonamides displace protein-bound sulphonylureas and increase the hypoglycaemic effect. They may also inhibit the metabolism of sulphonylureas. Lithium diminishes the hypoglycaemic effect of sulphonylureas. Glucose tolerance may deteriorate with the administration of a thiazide diuretic. Rifampicin reduces the hypoglycaemic effect of sulphonylureas because of the induction of metabolizing liver enzymes.

9. **A B D E**
   A high ethanol intake, and treatment with cholestyramine cause raised triglycerides due to increased hepatic synthesis and secretion, and treatment with propranolol also causes this because of reduced catabolism. Calcium antagonists do not have an adverse effect on serum lipid concentrations. Chronic renal failure causes raised triglycerides probably because of reduced hepatic and lipoprotein lipase activity.

10. **A C E**
    Zidovudine is a structural analogue of thymidine, and is rapidly absorbed by the oral route, although the oral bioavailability is only 60–65%. Zidovudine should not be given if the peripheral white cell count is less than 0.75×10^9/l. It has a half-life of about 1 hour.

11. A C E

Patients with acute intermittent porphyria should avoid the following drugs:

- alcohol
- barbiturates
- benzodiazepines
- chloroquine
- grisofulvin
- methyldopa
- oral contraceptives
- phenytoin
- rifampicin
- sulphonamides
- sulphonylureas

12. A B D E

Aspirin potentiates the action of oral hypoglycaemics, warfarin, non-steroidal anti-inflammatory drugs, steroids and alcohol.

13. A B C D

Aminoglycosides and tetracyclines have a direct nephrotoxic effect and may cause an acute tubular necrosis. Penicillins, sulphonamides, tetracycline, rifampicin and streptomycin may cause an acute interstitial nephritis.

14. B D E

The following sympathomimetic amines should be avoided in patients on monoamine oxidase inhibitor therapy: tricyclic antidepressants, amphetamines, pethidine, barbiturates and L-dopa. The resulting interacting effect includes the risk of a hypertensive crisis, CNS excitation and hyperpyrexia, and prolongation of the action of interacting drugs.

15. A B E

Other drugs associated with photosensitivity include sulphonamides, griseofulvin, nalidixic acid, thiazide diuretics and both oestrogens and progesterones.

16. A B D E

Rifampicin (also phenytoin, carbamazepine, phenobarbitone, isoniazid, benzodiazepines, chloramphenicol and griseofulvin) reduces the contraceptive action due to enzyme induction. Chloral hydrate may transiently enhance the anticoagulant effect of warfarin. Monoamine oxidase inhibitors may increase the effect of L-dopa. Digoxin toxicity is enhanced by beta blockers.

17. A B D E

Intrahepatic cholestatic jaundice (and hepatitis) may be caused by phenothiazines, tricyclic antidepressants, non-steroidal anti-inflammatory drugs, sulphonylureas, rifampicin, erythromycin and sulphonamides. Norethandrolone and oral contraceptives cause cholestasis alone. Repeated administration of halothane, isoniazid, pyrazinamide, rifampicin, monoamine oxidase inhibitors, methyldopa and anticonvulsants may cause an acute hepatitis 2–3 weeks after exposure. Carbon tetrachloride is a hepatotoxin.

18. B D E

Phenytoin has a narrow therapeutic range, and the relationship between dose and plasma concentration is non-linear. The long-term effects of phenytoin may include a folate deficiency and megaloblastic anaemia. Phenytoin will displace iodine from its protein-binding sites.

19. B D E

Therapeutic monitoring of plasma drug concentrations is used for drugs with a narrow therapeutic range (e.g. lithium), or which show dose-dependent kinetics (e.g. phenytoin). Drug level monitoring is available for:

antiarrhythmics – procainamide and quinidine
antibiotics – aminoglycosides
anticonvulsants – phenobarbitone, phenytoin and carbamazepine
digoxin
others – aminophylline, lithium

20. B C E

Aspirin may have an adverse effect in the second and third trimester: it impairs platelet function and increases the risk of haemorrhage. Phenytoin is associated with congenital malformations and screening is advised. The main effects of corticosteroids in pregnancy are in the second and third trimester, and may include fetal and neonatal adrenal suppression. Fansidar has a possible teratogenic risk because pyrimethamine is a folate antagonist. Other teratogenic drugs include:

alcohol – fetal alcohol syndrome
androgens – virilization
cytotoxic agents – fetal malformations
diethylstilboestrol – adenocarcinoma of vagina
radioactive iodine – fetal thyroid damage
warfarin – fetal warfarin syndrome

21. A B D E

The antidote for iron poisoning is desferrioxamine; for paracetamol is N-acetyl cysteine or methionine; for morphine or other opiates is naloxone, an oral opiate antagonist; and for cyanide is sodium thiosulphate or cobalt edetate.

22. B C D E

Digoxin toxicity depends on both the plasma concentration of the drugs and on the sensitivity of the myocardium, which is often increased in heart disease. Hypokalaemia predisposes to toxicity, therefore diuretics used with digoxin should either be potassium sparing or should be given with potassium supplements. Verapamil, beta-blockers, hypercalcaemia, quinidine and amiodarone all enhance digoxin toxicity.

23. A B E

Other drugs associated with gynaecomastia include cimetidine, methyldopa, phenothiazines, tricyclic antidepressants and cytotoxic agents.

24. A B C E

Other drugs associated with galactorrhoea include L-dopa, metoclopramide, cimetidine, benzodiazepines and oestrogens.

25. A B C D E

Side effects of ergotamine include vomiting and abdominal pain. Repeated high dose may cause ergotism with gangrene and confusion. As with methysergide, pleural and peritoneal fibrosis may occur with excessive use.

26. A C D E

Drugs to be avoided in renal failure include:

anti-infectives, e.g. tetracyclines, nitrofurantoin, amphotericin B
aspirin and non-steroidal anti-inflammatory drugs
lithium
narcotic analgesics
potassium-sparing diuretics and potassium supplements

Drugs which require a dose reduction in renal failure include:

anti-infectives, e.g. penicillin, aminoglycosides, cephalosporins, suphonamides, vancomycin, metronidazole
methyldopa, digoxin, procainamide and disopyramide
others, e.g. chlorpropamide, insulin and H_2-antagonists

27. D E

Dopamine acts on the beta-1 receptors in cardiac muscle. It increases contractility with little effect on rate, and is therefore used in cardiogenic shock. The dose of dopamine is critical since low doses inducevasodilatation and increase renal perfusion, whereas higher doses (>5μg/kg/min) lead to vasoconstriction and may exacerbate heart failure.

28. A D

Glyceryl trinitrate is a potent coronary vasodilator, but its principal benefit follows from a reduction in venous return which reduces left ventricular work. Unwanted effects include a throbbing headache, flushing, postural hypotension and tachycardia. Isoprenaline is an unselective inotropic sympathomimetic cardiac stimulant, and increases both heart rate and contractility. It is now used only as a short-term emergency treatment of bradycardia or heart block.

29. A C E

Agents causing direct hepatotoxicity are tetracycline, carbon tetrachloride, methotrexate, azathioprine, paracetamol and aflatoxin.

30. A B C D

Other agents causing peripheral neuropathy include:

streptomycin, metronidazole, nalidixic acid, chloramphenicol
oral hypoglycaemics, e.g. sulphonylureas
anti-TB agents, e.g. isoniazid, ethambutol
phenelzine and tricyclic antidepressants

31. A B E

Other agents causing pulmonary fibrosis include nitrofurantoin, sulphasalazine, practolol, amiodarone and prolonged high-dose oxygen.

32. A C D

Drugs which may cause aplastic anaemia include:

anti-arrhythmics, e.g. quinidine and procainamide
antibiotics, e.g. chloramphenicol, sulphonamides, methicillin, ampicillin, cotrimoxazole
anti-convulsants, e.g. carbamazepine, phenytoin
anti-malarials, e.g. pyrimethamine, chloroquine
anti-rheumatic agents, e.g. gold salts, penicillamine
anti-thyroid agents, e.g. carbimazole
cytotoxic agents
diuretics, e.g. thiazides and frusemide
oral hypoglycaemics, e.g. sulphonylureas
phenothiazines
tricyclic antidepressants

33. A B E

Other drugs that may cause erythema nodosum include salicylates and phenylbutazone, sulphonylureas, e.g. chlorpropamide, oral contraceptives and gold salts.

34. A B C E

Diarrhoea, with or without abdominal pain, is the most common side effect of oral therapy with gold salts, and may respond to bulking agents or temporary reductions in dosage. Severe reactions occur in up to 5% of patients, and include aplastic anaemia, proteinuria, mouth ulcers, pulmonary fibrosis, peripheral neuritis, hepatotoxicity with cholestatic jaundice, and alopecia.

35. A B C D E

Other long-term effects of phenytoin therapy include hypersensitivity reactions, rashes, SLE syndrome, lymphadenopathy and slurred speech.

36. B E

Hypersensitivity reactions may also involve urticaria, angio-oedema and anaphylaxis. Osteoporosis and, rarely, alopecia may occur with long-term use.

37. A B C D E

'Oxidant' drugs to avoid with G6PDH deficiency:

analgesics, e.g. aspirin and phenacetin
anti-infectives, e.g. chloramphenicol, sulphonamides, nitrofurantoin, dapsone and cotrimoxazole
anti-malarials, e.g. chloroquine, primaquine and quinine
others, e.g. probencid and quinidine

38. A B E

The use of ergometrine for acute attacks of migraine may be associated with peripheral vasospasm. Repeated high doses may cause ergotism with gangrene and confusion. Beta-blockers are associated with coldness of the extremities and Raynaud's phenomenon, although this may be less with those with intrinsic sympathomimetic activity (ISA), e.g. oxyprenolol, pindolol and acebutolol. Other adverse effects associated with clonidine include dry mouth, sedation, depression, fluid retention, bradycardia and impotence. Sudden withdrawal may cause a hypertensive crisis.

39. A B E

Drugs that may cause hyperuricaemia include thiazide and loop diuretics, pyrazinamide, ethambutol, cytotoxic agents and alcohol. Low dose aspirin (not high dose) is associated with hyperuricaemia.

40. A B C D

See answer to Question 26 above.

41. A C D E

Profound hypokalaemia may develop rapidly following overdosage with theophylline and related drugs. Forced alkaline diuresis and charcoal haemoperfusion are the treatment options for the small minority of patients with very severe barbiturate poisoning who fail to improve despite supportive care. Acetylcysteine may protect the liver if given within 10–12 hours of ingestion of paracetamol.

42. B C D

Other interacting drugs that may decrease the effect of oral contraceptives due to enzyme induction include phenobarbitone, isoniazid, benzodiazepines, chloramphenicol and griseofulvin.

43. A B C D E

Other characteristic side effects of these cytotoxic agents include:

methotrexate – hepatotoxicity, pneumonitis and encephalopathy
busulphan – aplastic anaemia and skin pigmentation
vincristine – joint pain, paralytic ileus, peripheral neuropathy and hyponatraemia
cyclophosphamide – skin pigmentation

44. C D E

Other drugs that may cause photosensitivity include:

anti-infectives, e.g. sulphonamides and tetracyclines
oestrogens and progesterones
phenothiazines
thiazide diuretics

45. A B D E

Plasma concentrations are not a useful index of efficacy, therefore routine monitoring is unhelpful. Other side effects of sodium valproate include ataxia, transient hair loss, oedema, thrombocytopenia, amenorrhoea, leucopenia and gynaecomastia.

46. C D E

Interferons are naturally occurring proteins with a variety of effects on cell mediated immune function including: (i) suppression of viral replication; (ii) anti-tumour activity; (iii) activation of macrophages and natural killer cells. Alfa interferon has shown some anti-tumour effect in certain lymphomas and solid tumours. Side-effects are dose-related and may include influenza-type symptoms, lethargy and depression. Myelosuppression may also occur, particularly granulocytopenia.

47. A B C D

Other potential side effects of thiazides include hypokalaemia, hypomagnesaemia, hyperuricaemia, hyperglycaemia, acute urinary retention, pancreatitis, inhibition of calcium excretion, rashes and thrombocytopenia.

INDEX

Page numbers refer to the page on which relevant *questions* appear. The word indexed may appear only in the *answer* to the question.

Other MRCP Part 1 Revision Books available from PasTest today!

✔MCQs Related to the Oxford Textbook of Medicine: 3rd ed.
350 new MCQs related to the 1995 Oxford Textbook of Medicine. All answers include appropriate OTM page references - this new edition includes explanatory teaching notes.

✔Medicine International Book 3 & Book 4
350 MCQs related to the monthly journal Medicine International. All answers and teaching notes include Medicine International page references. Both books contain different questions.

✔MRCP Part 1 MCQ Revision Book: 3rd ed.
300 MCQs arranged by subject plus one Mock Exam. Questions are similar to the official College exam. Basic sciences well represented.

✔MRCP Part 1 Practice Exams: 2nd ed.
A new edition of a *best seller* with 5 MCQ papers (300 MCQs). Strong emphasis on basic sciences questions and favourite RCP topics.

✔MRCP Part 1 MCQs with Individual Subject Summaries
200 exam-based MCQs arranged by subject. Correct answers with informative subject summaries provide revision synopses for important exam topics.

✔Explanations to the RCP Past Papers Green Book 1990
Correct answers and expert teaching notes related to the RCP green book of actual MRCP past exam questions.

✔Explanations to the RCP Blue Book 1982-3 (mail order only)
Correct answers and expert teaching notes related to the RCP blue book of actual MRCP past exam questions.

MRCP Part 1 Paediatrics:

✔MRCP Part 1 Paediatric MCQ Revision Book
Over 300 new MCQs based on recent exam questions, plus one complete MCQ practice exam of 60 questions, correct answers and expanded teaching notes.

✔Explanations to the Royal College Red Booklet (mail order only)
Answers related to the RCP book of sample paediatric questions.

PTO ➧

MRCP Part 1 Pocket Books:

✔Pocket Book 1: Cardiology, Respiratory Medicine

✔Pocket Book 2: Neurology, Psychiatry

✔Pocket Book 3: Gastroenterology, Endocrinology, Renal

✔Pocket Book 4: Rheum, Haem, Infectious diseases
Each pocket sized book contains 100 MCQs on favourite Membership topics. Basic sciences well represented, correct answers and detailed teaching notes

Multiple Choice Questions on Disk:

✔Membership at your Finger-tips: MCQs on Disk
This unique software gives you the vital practice you need to succeed. With over 600 exam based MCQs, accompanied by answers and comprehensive teaching notes prepared by experts in the field, this product is an invaluable component to any successful revision strategy.

✔Membership at your Finger-tips: Demonstration Disk (FREE)
An opportunity to trial this indispensable software before you purchase it.

Contact us today for full details of our complete range of books and courses.

PasTest, Freepost, Knutsford, Cheshire WA16 7BR
Tel: 01565 755226 ● Fax: 01565 650264